PEDIATRIC PEARLS
The Handbook of Practical Pediatrics

Pediatric Pearls

The Handbook of Practical Pediatrics

Beryl J. Rosenstein, M.D.
Professor of Pediatrics
The Johns Hopkins University School of Medicine
Baltimore, Maryland

Patricia D. Fosarelli, M.D.
Assistant Professor of Pediatrics
The Johns Hopkins University School of Medicine
Baltimore, Maryland

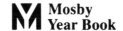
Mosby
Year Book

St. Louis   Baltimore   Boston   Chicago   London   Philadelphia   Sydney   Toronto

A Year Book Medical Publishers imprint of Mosby–Year Book, Inc.

Mosby–Year Book, Inc.
11830 Westline Industrial Drive
St. Louis, MO 63146

4 5 6 7 8 9 0 PX 93 92 91

Library of Congress Cataloging-in-Publication Data

Rosenstein, Beryl J.
Pediatrics Pearls: The Handbook of Practical Pediatrics/
Beryl J. Rosenstein, Patricia D. Fosarelli.
p. cm
Includes bibliographies and index.
ISBN 0-8151-7396-2
1. Pediatrics—Handbooks, manuals, etc.
I. Fosarelli, Patricia D. II. Title
{DNLM: 1. Pediatrics—Handbooks. WS 39 R815h}
RJ48/R67 1990
618.92—dc20
DNLM/DLC
for Library of Congress 89-9194 CIP

Sponsoring Editor: Nancy E. Chorpenning
Developmental Editor: Craig Pugh
Associate Managing Editor, Manuscript Services:
    Deborah Thorp
Production Project Coordinator: Carol Reynolds
Proofroom Manager: Barbara Kelly

Dedicated to the houseofficers of the Harriet Lane Home Service, past and present, who have been our best teachers as well as a constant source of support.

Acknowledgment

We are indebted to all of the chief residents of the Harriet Lane Home outpatient department who nurtured this project during its embryonic stages, and to Frank A. Oski, M.D., and Catherine DeAngelis, M.D., for their encouragement and support. We are grateful to a number of our colleagues at Hopkins who reviewed sections of the handbook. They include: Hoover Adger, George Dover, Anne Greene, Fred Heldrich, Alan Lake, Samuel Libber, Ambadas Pathak, Leslie Plotnick, Michael Repka, Saul Roskes, Kenneth Schuberth, Charles Shubin, Edward Sills, Harvey Singer, Timothy Townsend, Walter Tunnessen, Eileen Vining, Modena Wilson, Lawrence Wissow, and Kenneth Zahka. Lori Waugh provided excellent secretarial support. Her ability to decipher and decode our rough drafts was a source of constant relief and amazement. We thank Richard S. Ross, M.D., Dean of the Johns Hopkins University School of Medicine and Robert M. Heyssel, M.D., President of The Johns Hopkins Hospital, for allowing us to use The Johns Hopkins Hospital logo on the cover, especially in this 100th anniversary year of the medical institutions. Last, but certainly not least, we thank Nancy Chorpenning, Craig Pugh, and their colleagues at Year Book Medical Publishers for all of their editorial, organizational, and moral support in bringing this project to completion.

BERYL J. ROSENSTEIN, M.D.
PATRICIA D. FOSARELLI, M.D.

PREFACE

For many years, The Johns Hopkins Hospital pediatric residents have regularly referred to their "Therapeutic Shorts," as early editions of this book were called, during their rotations, especially in the emergency room and outpatient clinics. Many medical students reported that they learned much of the practical aspects of pediatric diagnosis and therapy from it. "Therapeutic Shorts" was never considered to be a replacement of its more famous relative, *The Harriet Lane Handbook;* instead, it was considered a supplement to *The Harriet Lane Handbook* with "pearls of wisdom" in diagnosis and management of the more common pediatric problems.

Even though this present text has been much expanded from those early editions of "Therapeutic Shorts," we still consider it to be a companion to *The Harriet Lane Handbook*. We have added new sections and expanded old ones in the preparation of this book, yet there is very little overlap with *The Harriet Lane Handbook*, since the purposes of the books are very different. *The Harriet Lane Handbook* is a compendium of information necessary for students and houseofficers to have at their fingertips if they are to function optimally. It is a quick reference to use in the middle of the night or on a busy service when other texts are unavailable and a visit to the library is impossible. *Pediatric Pearls: The Handbook of Practical Pediatrics* is meant to be a guide to the INITIAL management of common pediatric conditions. It is not meant to be exhaustive, but instead to be a portable body of practical advice on how to approach a problem from initial assessment, differential diagnosis, and diagnostic tests, to therapy options. As such, its usefulness is not limited to houseofficers and students, but it will be helpful to any professional who cares for children, especially those on the "front lines." We hope this book will well serve both its readers and the children they care for.

Beryl J. Rosenstein, M.D.
Patricia D. Fosarelli, M.D.

Contents

Abbreviations

A-V	Arteriovenous
Abd	Abdominal
ABG	Arterial blood gas
AGN	Acute glomerulonephritis
AgNO$_3$	Silver nitrate
ALT	Alanine transferase
ALTE	Apparent life-threatening event
ANA	Antinuclear antibody
ASA	Acetylsalicylic acid
ASO	Antistreptolysin-O
AST	Aspartate transferase
bid	Twice a day
BP	Blood pressure
BPD	Bronchopulmonary dysplasia
bpm	Beats per minute
BUN	Blood urea nitrogen
C	Centigrade
C+S	Culture and sensitivity
C-spine	Cervical spine
Ca	Calcium
cbc	Complete blood count
CC	Cubic centimeters
CDC	Centers for Disease Control
CDH	Congenital dislocation of hip
CF	Cystic fibrosis
CHF	Congestive heart failure
CIE	Counter immunoelectrophoresis
cm	Centimeter
CMV	Cytomegalovirus
CNS	Central nervous system
CO	Carbon monoxide
Col	Colonies
CPK	Creatine phosphokinase

(Continued)

CPR	Cardiopulmonary resuscitation
CRP	C-reactive protein
CSF	Cerebrospinal fluid
CT	Computed tomography
CV	Cardiovascular
CVA	Costovertebral angle
CXR	Chest x-ray
d	Day
D/C	Discontinue
D5W	5% Dextrose in water
DEA	Drug Enforcement Agency
DIC	Disseminated intravascular coagulation
diff	Differential
DKA	Diabetic ketoacidosis
dl	Deciliter
DMT	Dimethyltryptamine
DTP	Diphtheria-tetanus-pertussis
DTR	Deep tendon reflex
Dx	Diagnosis
EBV	Epstein-Barr virus
ECG	Electrocardiogram
EDTA	Edetate disodium
EEG	Electroencephalogram
ELISA	Enzyme-linked-immunosorbent assay
EM	Erythema multiforme
ENT	Ear, nose and throat
EOS	Eosinophils
ER	Emergency room
ESR	Erythrocyte sedimentation rate
ET	Endotracheal
ETT	Endotracheal tube
F	Fahrenheit
F/U	Follow-up
FB	Foreign body
Fe	Iron
FEP	Free erythrocyte protoporphyrin
FHx	Family history
FSH	Follicle stimulating hormone
FTAb-ABS	Fluorescent treponemal antibody absorption test
FTT	Failure to thrive
Fx	Fracture

(Continued)

G-	Gram negative
GC	Gonococcal
GE	Gastroesophageal
GER	Gastroesophageal reflux
G6PD	Glucose-6-phosphate dehydrogenase
GI	Gastrointestinal
gm	Gram
GU	Genitourinary
GYN	Gynecology
h	Hour
H/O	History of
H2O2	Hydrogen peroxide
HBIG	Hepatitis B immune globulin
HC	Head circumference
HCO3	Bicarbonate
Hct	Hematocrit
HDCV	Human diploid cell vaccine
HEENT	Head, eyes, ears, nose and throat
Hg	Mercury
Hgb	Hemoglobin
HIV	Human immunodeficiency virus
hpf	High power field
HR	Heart rate
hr	Hour
hs	At bedtime
HSP	Henoch-Schönlein purpura
HSV	Herpes simplex virus
HUS	Hemolytic-uremic syndrome
Hx	History
I + D	Incision and drainage
ICP	Intracranial pressure
IDDM	Insulin-dependent diabetes mellitus
IFA	Immunofluorescent antibody
IM	Intramuscular
ISG	Immune serum globulin
iu	International unit
IV	intravenous
IVP	Intravenous pyelogram
JRA	Juvenile rheumatoid arthritis
K	Potassium
Kcal	Kilo calories

(Continued)

KCL	Potassium chloride
KOH	Potassium hydroxide
KS	Ketosteroid
KV	Killivolt
LATS	Long-acting thyroid stimulating hormone
LDH	Lactic dehydrogenase
LFT's	Liver function tests
LH	Luteinizing hormone
LP	Lumbar puncture
LSD	Lysergic acid diethylamide
MAX	Maximum
MCHC	Mean corpuscular hemoglobin concentration
MCV	Mean corpuscular volume
MDA	Methylenedioxyamphetamine
mEq	Milliequivalent
mg	Milligram
min	Minute
MLNS	Mucocutaneous lymph node syndrome
mm	Millimeter
MMR	Measles-mumps-rubella
mo	Months
NaHCO3	Sodium bicarbonate
NB	Note well
Neg	Negative
NG	Nasogastric
NH4	Ammonia
NIDDM	Non-insulin-dependent diabetes mellitus
NP	Nasopharyngeal
NPO	Nothing by mouth
O2	Oxygen
OGES	Oral glucose-electrolyte solution
OM	Otitis media
OPV	Oral polio vaccine (Sabin)
OR	Operating room
OTC	Over the counter
OZ	Ounce
P	Pulse = HR (Heart rate)
PA	Posterioanterior
Pb	Lead
PCP	Phencyclidine
PE	Physical examination

(Continued)

PID	Pelvic inflammatory disease (salpingitis)
PMI	Point of maximal impulse
PMN's`	Polymorphonuclear cells
po	By mouth
PO_4	Phosphate
PRN	As needed
pt	Patient
PVC	Premature ventricular contraction
q	every
q x h	Every "x" hours
qd	Once a day
qid	Four times a day
qtt	Drops
R/O	Rule out
RAI	Radioactive iodine uptake
RBC	Red blood cell
REM	Rapid eye movement
RIG	Rabies immune globulin
RMSF	Rocky Mountain spotted fever
RR	Respiratory rate
RSV	Respiratory syncytial virus
Rx	Treat
S/P	Status post
s/sx	Signs/Symptoms
SBE	Subacute bacterial endocarditis
SCFE	Slipped capital femoral epiphysis
SJS	Stevens-Johnson syndrome
SIADH	Syndrome of inappropriate antidiuretic hormone
SIDS	Sudden infant death syndrome
Sig	Directions
SLE	Systemic lupus eythematosis
SOM	Serous otitis media
SQ	Subcutaneous
SS	Sickle cell
STD's	Sexually transmitted diseases
STS	Serologic test for syphilis
T	Temperature
T+A	Tonsillectomy and adenoidectomy
T/C	Throat culture
T3	Triiodothyronine
T4	Free thyroxine

(Continued)

TAC	Tetracaine, adrenaline, and cocaine
TB	Tuberculosis
TCA	Tricyclic antidepressant
TEF	Tracheo-esophageal fistula
THC	Tetrahydrocannabinol
TIBC	Total iron-binding capacity
tid	Three times a day
TM	Tympanic membrane
TMP/SMZ	Trimethoprim-sulfamethoxazole
TRICH	Trichomonas
TSH	Thyroid-stimulating hormone
tsp	Teaspoon
Tx	Treatment
u	Unit
U/A	Urinalysis
URI	Upper respiratory infection
US	Ultrasound
UTI	Urinary tract infection
V-P	Ventriculo-peritoneal
VCUG	Voiding cystourethrogram
VGE	Viral gastroenteritis
VZIG	Varicella-Zoster immune globulin
w/u	Workup
WBC	White blood cell
yr	Year
ZnPP	Zinc protoporphyrin
~	Approximately
≤	Equal to or less than
≥	Equal to or greater than
µg	Microgram

GENERAL APPROACH
TO THE PATIENT

A. History

1. A careful, pertinent, and thorough history is an essential first step in understanding any patient's problem(s). In addition to the chief complaint and the present illness, explore past history, medications, immunizations, hospitalizations, prior surgery, transfusions, previous major illnesses and accidents, recent exposures, general prior health, family history, social situation, and sources of medical care. Record this information in such a way that it will be both available and useful in the future. Be sure to talk to the person most knowledgeable about the patient's history.

2. Be alert for "the hidden diagnosis" (i.e., the patient's or family's presenting complaint may have little or nothing to do with the actual problem). Try to determine what is really troubling the patient and/or family. Open-ended questions might be especially helpful in this regard.

   Example: Chief Complaint = stomach pains.
   Actual Diagnosis = school phobia, sexual abuse, etc.

3. Include in history:
   a. Patient's address and phone number (or nearest phone).
   b. Parent's or guardian's name.
   c. Name and address of private doctor or clinic where patient usually receives medical care.

B. **Physical Exam (PE)**

   1. Obtain weight, length, and vital signs (T, P, RR for all age groups and BP for children and adolescents), and HC (if appropriate, such as during a visit for an infant/toddler).

   2. PE should include pertinent positives and negatives. Do not limit exam to the organ system which is the basis for the chief complaint.

C. **Laboratory**

   Order only those tests which will affect management. It is imperative to follow-up on the results. A multi-million dollar workup is not indicated every time a diagnosis is uncertain.

MANAGING "ANY DOCTOR" CALLS: MEDICINE BY TELEPHONE

D. General Principles

1. Identify yourself.
2. Request identification of the child, caller, and the caller's relationship to the child.
3. Ascertain the child's age and an approximation of his weight.
4. Listen to the parent's story.
5. When asking questions, wait for the answer to one question before going on to the next one.
6. Remain courteous and calm (even if the parent is neither).
7. Avoid ambiguous or medical terms that might confuse the parent.

8. Identify the child's problem to your satisfaction before rendering advice; plainly state what you believe the problem to be.
9. If the child is not to be seen, explain why not, and give the parent specific therapies to try as well as advice on what to do if the therapies fail.
10. Instruct the parent on the symptoms that are part of the natural course of the illness and those that are a warning that the child is worsening. Indicate which symptoms warrant medical attention.
11. Ask the parent to repeat any instructions you have given and ask whether there are any questions.
12. Encourage the parent to call back if s/he has questions or the child's condition changes.
13. Follow-up on any child that concerns you. (Do not depend on the parent to call back.) If the family has no phone, obtain the phone number of a relative/friend.

E. Special Principles for the Most Common Problems Presenting by Phone (from *Pediatric Primary Care*, 3rd ed., DeAngelis, C., Little, Brown and Co., 1984, pp. 68-70).

1. Respiratory Complaints
   a. Does the child have a cold? Is it getting better or worse? In what way?
   b. Has the child had a fever? How high?
   c. What medicines (how much, for how long, and how often) have been used for the fever and for the cold?
   d. Does he have a cough? Does he vomit with it?
   e. Is his nose runny? What color is the nasal discharge?
   f. Does he seem to breathe more noisily than usual?
   g. When he breathes, can you see his ribs?
   h. Is any area of his body blue?
   i. Are his nostrils moving with each breath?

    j. Can you count his breaths for me? (If the parent does not have a watch with a second hand, she can count out loud, and you can time the breaths.)

    k. Does he have a hoarse cry or barky cough?

    l. Does he have a rash?

    m. Is he vomiting or having diarrhea?

    n. How is he eating, sleeping, and acting?

    o. What is he doing now?

2. Fever
   a. Did you take the infant's temperature, or did he just feel warm?
   b. What was the temperature? Rectal or oral?
   c. Has he been given fever medicine? Which one, how much, and how often? When was the last dose?
   d. Does his fever seem to come down with the medicine?
   e. What else have you tried to make him better?
   f. What other signs of illness does he have (respiratory problems, rash, etc.)?
   g. How is he acting, sleeping, eating?
   h. Has he received a shot? What kind? When?
   i. Does he seem to be in pain? How so?
   j. Are contacts ill?

3. Dermatologic Problems
   a. How long has the child had the rash, and where did it first appear?
   b. Where is it now? Is it on the palms and soles?
   c. What color is the rash, and how large are the individual spots?
   d. Can you feel the rash as well as see it?
   e. Does it disappear with pressure?
   f. Does any part of the rash have blisters or crusts?
   g. Does the rash itch, burn, or hurt?
   h. Has he had a similar rash in the past?
   i. Has he been around anyone else with a similar rash?
   j. What other signs of illness does he have?

    k. How is he eating, sleeping, and playing?

    l. Does he have a fever?

4. Trauma

    a. What kind of injury did the child sustain (fall, laceration, burn, bite, etc.)? How and when did it occur? To which body part was the injury sustained?

    b. If the child struck his head, did he lose consciousness, vomit, or seize after the episode? How is he acting now? If he injured another body part, is he using it normally now? What has the parent done?

    c. If the child sustained a laceration, is he still bleeding? How large is the laceration? Is the blood bright red and spurting? What has the parent done to stop the bleeding? What is the child doing now? When was his last tetanus shot?

    d. If the child was burned, what body part was burned? How large an area is involved? Is there an area of redness, or are there blisters? Have the blisters broken? Does he complain of pain at the burn site? What has the parent done for the burn? How is the child acting? When was his last tetanus shot?

    e. If the child was bitten, what bit him? If a dog bit him, is the dog known to the family? Has it been behaving abnormally? Has it had its shots? Was the dog provoked? If a wild animal bit him, what type of animal was it? When was the child's last tetanus shot? What has the parent done for him? How does the area look, and how is the child acting? Do they have the animal?

5. Gastrointestinal Complaints

    a. Is the child having diarrhea, vomiting, or both?

    b. How long has this been occurring?

    c. If the child is vomiting, is he merely coughing up phlegm, spitting up after feeding, or actually vomiting?

d. When does the vomiting occur in relation to meals?
e. Can he take certain foods without vomiting? Which ones?
f. Can he drink anything without vomiting?
g. Has he accidentally ingested a household product or a medication?
h. Does the vomitus come out with force, or effortlessly?
i. Does he seem hungry or in pain?
j. How many bowel movements today? Yesterday?
k. How many times has he thrown up today? Yesterday?
l. Is the vomitus or stool red or green?
m. What does the stool look like? Does it have any formed elements in it?
n. Is the child on any medication?
o. What has the parent done for the illness (including dietary and medicinal regimens)?
p. Is the illness getting better or worse?
q. Is his mouth wet?
r. Has he been urinating the usual number of times and amounts?
s. What other signs of illness does he have (rash, respiratory symptoms, etc.)?
t. Has he had a fever? How high was it?
u. How is he sleeping?
v. How is his appetite for foods and liquids?
w. What liquids and foods has the mother given him today? How were they tolerated?
x. How is his activity?
y. Do any of his contacts have similar complaints?
z. What is he doing now?

III.THERAPEUTICS

F. Medications

1. Consider whether the drug is really indicated; what therapeutic effect to expect; side effects (may differ according to age of patient); half-life; dosage; cost (use generic when possible); interactions with other drugs (erythromycin and theophylline); risk of poisoning.

2. Consider the most appropriate form of administration (tablet, capsule, liquid, suppository, etc.).

3. Consider frequency and periodicity of administration ("qid" is generally 8 am-12 noon-4 pm-8 pm, while "q6h" is 8 am-2 pm-8 pm-2 am). Simplify regimens as much as possible, and make them convenient with school, sleep, etc.

4. Arrange to follow blood levels where necessary (e.g., anticonvulsants and theophylline).

5. Consider compliance of patient and family. Compliance decreases as number of medications increases and if specified times for administration are inconvenient.

6. Teach your patient about the medication's indications, effects, side effects, how to accurately measure and administer it, and how to prevent inadvertent overdosing.

   a. Have patient or parent repeat what you have told them.

   b. Special instructions should always be written out.

   c. Explain to parents that the medication must be taken for full course, even if symptoms disappear in two days.

7. Document and report adverse drug effects.

G. Prescriptions

1. Be sure your patient will be able to get the prescription filled.

2. Write legibly. Not only is it inconsiderate to write illegibly, it is potentially dangerous if prescriptions are filled incorrectly. Use only standard abbreviations.
3. Include all pertinent information.
   a. Patient's name, address, age.
   b. Name of drug, form (tablet, liquid, capsule, etc.), dosage or concentration (500 mg tablet, 500 mg/5 cc, 250 mg/5 cc).
   c. Amount dispensed: i.e., number of tablets, amount of liquid (round off to nearest 10 cc if applicable).
   d. Directions: (Sig:) amount, frequency, route, and duration (e.g., 5 cc every 4 hours po x 7 days). Do not use teaspoon measures.
   e. Indication if refill is necessary, how many times, or no refill.
   f. Don't forget your signature and DEA number if controlled substance is prescribed.
4. Include all prescription data (name of drug, form, dosing regimen, and amount dispensed) in patient's medical record.

H. Counseling the Patient and Family

1. *Essential* for physician and patient rapport. Improves communication and understanding of illness; improves compliance with follow-up and medication; alleviates fears and misconceptions; prevents mismanagement at home; patient and family know what to expect and when to return if certain signs or symptoms develop. Nurses can teach temperature measurement and go over with patient/parents what has been told to them.
2. In general, it is better to contact the family for telephone follow-up. Arrange a time and number where they can be reached. Keep track of patients in need of telephone contact.

REFERENCES

1. Sackett DL; and Haynes RB (eds): *Compliance with Therapeutic Regimens*. The Johns Hopkins University Press, Baltimore, 1976.
2. Weintraub M, et al.:Compliance as a Determinant of Serum Digoxin Concentrations. *JAMA 224*: 481-485, 1973.
3. Frances PHN; Korsch BM; and Moriss MJ: Gaps in Doctor-Patient Communication. Patients response to Medical Advice. *NEJM 280*: 535-540, 1969.
4. Charney E: Patient-Doctor Communication. Implications for the Clinician. *PCNA 19*: 2, p. 263, 1972.
5. Dawson KP and Jamieson A: Value of Blood Phenytoin Estimation in Management of Childhood Epilepsy. *Arch Dis Child 46*: 386-388, 1971.
6. Matter ME, et. al.: Inadequacies in the Pharmacologic Management of Ambulatory Children. *J Pediatr 87*: 137-141, 1975.

2

PEDIATRIC CARDIOPULMONARY RESUSCITATION

A. The Alphabet of Resuscitation (A, B, C, D, E)

Remember: Most pediatric arrests are primarily pulmonary events.

<u>A</u>irway: Airway obstruction is commonly the precipitating event in cardiopulmonary arrest of a child.

Clear oropharynx of secretions, vomitus (suctioning or careful finger sweep); should not be done blindly.

Open the airway using the chin-lift or jaw-thrust technique. In the traumatized child, <u>do not</u> hyperextend the neck. Rather, maintain in-line traction. An oral airway may be inserted to avoid obstruction of airway by the tongue. The tip of the airway should just approximate the angle of the mandible.

<u>B</u>reathe: With the exception of total airway obstruction as occurs with foreign body aspiration, any child may be effectively ventilated via bag and mask. This technique should be utilized until endotracheal tube placement is feasible. Watch

chest for good expansion, and note improvement in perfusion and pulses. If bag-valve-mask technique is insufficient, or if adequate and spontaneous respirations are not able to be maintained, the patient should be intubated. You may need muscle relaxants to intubate (discussed below). Assess patient after intubation for equal breath sounds bilaterally and for adequacy of ventilation/perfusion. Pulse oximetry can be very helpful.
Endotracheal tube size:
Newborn 3.0-3.5 mm (internal diameter)

$$\text{Tube diameter (mm)} = \frac{\text{age in yr} + 16}{4}$$

ET tube size approximates diameter of patient's little finger.

Circulation: • Make sure a firm board is under chest for effective closed-chest cardiac massage.
• 1 breath/4-5 compressions (ratio remains the same regardless of age or size).
• Time of compression = Time uncompressed for best cardiac output.

	Infant	Child	Adult
Compression (Rate/min)	100	80	60
Depth of compression (in.)	1/2-1	1-1 1/2	1 1/2-2
Ventilation (rate/min)	20	16	12

• Synchronize compression with respirations (ventilate as compression is released).
• Compression should be applied evenly over the midsternum. This is the point where the transnipple line intersects the sternum.

• Check efficacy of CPR.

Palpate peripheral pulses while pumping (femoral, brachial, carotid).

Assess perfusion.

Assess ventilation.

Assess pupil reactivity.

<u>D</u>rugs: It is essential to know the indications/effects/dosages of a few "first-line" resuscitation drugs. These are listed here and in the *Harriet Lane Handbook*.

You do not have to wait for an ECG or ABG before giving medicines.

Establish good vascular access ASAP. Whenever possible, a central intravenous site should be obtained. Peripheral sites may be inadequate for getting drugs into the central circulation. If a percutaneous venous line cannot be established quickly (within 2 minutes), perform a cutdown or place an intraosseous infusion needle.

Remember: Four drugs may be given via endotracheal tube.

These are: Lidocaine
Atropine
Naloxone
Epinephrine

Drug	Indication	Effect	Dose
Epinephrine	Asystole, Ventricular fibrillation	+Inotropic +chronotropic May convert fine ventricular fibrillation to coarse ventricular fibrillation-enhance chance of successful cardioversion. Less effective in presence of severe metabolic acidosis.	0.01 mg/kg of 1:10,000 dilution IV, (0.1 cc/kg) ETT, Intracardiac (intracardiac is last resort). Adult dose: 5–10 cc of 1:10,000 dilution; may repeat every 5 min.
NaHCO₃	Metabolic acidosis	↑ pH ↓ PCO₂ if not adequately ventilated.	1 mEq/kg IV slowly (1 cc/kg). Dilute standard 1 mEq/cc solution in half in newborn. Not effective if ventilation is inadequate. Adult dose: 1–2 amps (44 mEq/amp). Note: Be sure to clear IV line of NaHCO₃, as epinephrine and calcium are inactivated in alkaline solutions. Do not give via ETT.
Calcium 10% calcium chloride	Hypocalcemia Hyperkalemia	↑ Myocardial contractility counteracts K toxic effects. Bradycardia	10% Calcium chloride: 10–20 mg/kg or 0.1–0.25 cc/kg IV slowly. (Preferably through central line.) Adult dose: 10 cc. Remember to clear IV line of NaHCO₃. (NaHCO₃ + Ca = chalk.)
Atropine	Sinus bradycardia AV block Pre-Intubation	↓ Decreases vagal tone. Increases conduction through AV node.	0.02 mg/kg, minimum dose 0.15 mg, maximum dose 2 mg or 0.04 mg/kg (whichever is smaller). NOTE: Insufficient dose may cause paradoxical bradycardia. May be given by ETT or intraosseous.
Lidocaine	Ventricular fibrillation, ventricular tachycardia PVCs	↓ Automaticity and ectopic pacemakers.	Concentration 2% (20 mg/cc)1.0 mg/kg bolus IV (0.05 cc/kg) followed by continuous infusion of 10–50 micrograms/kg/min.

Other Drugs:

<u>Glucose:</u> Indicated if hypoglycemia is suspected. Best to begin continuous infusion of 10% dextrose. Bolus of D_{25} (2cc/kg) can be used but may result in rebound hypoglycemia if not followed by glucose infusion.

<u>Naloxone (Narcan):</u> Narcotic antidote. Dose 0.1 mg/kg every 2-3 min. May give a standard 2 mg dose to all ages.

<u>Dopamine:</u> Has many effects that are dose dependent. Expand intravascular volume in shock states secondary to hypovolemia before using dopamine.

Low Dose

1-7 µg/kg/min
  Increases renal blood flow

Moderate dose

7-20 µg/kg/min
  Increases cardiac output and BP

High dose

20-30 µg/kg/min
  Systemic vasoconstriction, decreases renal blood flow

Toxicity: Minimal at reasonable doses. Tachyarrhythmias and excessive BP. Avoid extravasation. Do not administer in alkaline solutions.

<u>Isoproterenol (Isuprel) Infusion:</u>

1) Status asthmaticus unresponsive to other measures

2) Decreased cardiac output unresponsive to digoxin and dopamine

Effects of isoproterenol on CV system: ↑HR, cardiac contractility.

Contraindicated in ischemic heart disease (including aortic stenosis). Starting dose: 0.02 µg/kg/min. Then increase to 0.10 µg/ kg/min. Further increase by 0.1

µg/kg/min every 15 minutes until improvement or toxicity. Usual maximum dose = 1.5 µg/kg/min.

Caution: When initiating isoproterenol infusions in asthmatics, establish 2 intravenous lines. Abrupt cessation of this drug (as occurs in IV dysfunction) may result in a quick return of severe bronchospasm. Also increases myocardial oxygen consumption, which may be dangerous if $PO_2 < 60$.

Toxicity: HR exceeds baseline by 40 bpm or dysrhythmia or S-T changes result.

Bretylium and Dobutamine: see *Harriet Lane Handbook;* PCNA 27(3):495, 1980.

ECG: Observe rhythms, complexes.

Defibrillation: Use in ventricular fibrillation. Place one paddle to right of upper sternum and below clavicle and the other paddle to the left of left nipple in anterior axillary line.

Dose: if <50kg:2 watt-seconds/kg
        if > 50 kg: 200 watt-seconds

If single shock not effective, continue cardiac massage, then repeat shock at double power. If not effective, give 3 shocks in succession, then:

epinephrine-shock-lidocaine-shock-bretylium-shock-bretylium-shock-lidocaine-shock.

B. Organization

1 person to direct and monitor (oversees whole procedure).

1 person to ventilate: Establish and maintain airway/NG tube.

1 person to administer cardiac massage.

1 or 2 people to establish venous access and draw blood studies.

1 person to draw up medications.

1 person to record medications, procedures, and pertinent occurrences.

1 "go-for" to get equipment, supplies, and other personnel if needed.

Total of 7-8 for arrest team. <u>Keep unnecessary people out of the way.</u>

C. **Muscle Relaxants**

1. Indications: Need to intubate in face of increased muscle tone seizures, or patients struggling with respiratory failure.

2. Drugs: First, atropine 0.02 mg/kg (minimum 0.15 mg) to block vagal effects of succinylcholine, then succinylcholine 1-2 mg/kg.

    a. Fasciculation with paralysis occurs within 30 seconds, lasts for few minutes.

    b. If worried about aspiration during fasciculation, e.g., recent meal, give defasciculating dose of pancuronium (Pavulon), 0.01 mg/kg, prior to succinylcholine; apply cricoid pressure while intubating.

    c. During elective intubation in conscious patient, may "obtund" with thiopental 2-4 mg/kg prior to succinylcholine (watch BP!).

3. WARNINGS! Succinylcholine contraindicated with hyperkalemic states, e.g., burns, glaucoma, penetrating ocular injuries, and at times in presence of severe increased intracranial pressure.

    a. Beware of muscle relaxants in patients with upper airway obstruction.

REFERENCES

1. Orlowski JP: *PCNA* 27:495, 1980.
2. Brill JE: Cardiopulmonary Resuscitation. *Pediatr Annals* 1986; 15:24-29.
3. Nugent S; Lavaruso L; and Rodgers M: Pharmacology and Use of Muscle Relaxants in Infants and Children. *J. Pediatr* 94:481, 1979.
4. Stanksi D and Sheiner L: Pharmacokinetics and Dynamics of Muscle Relaxants. *Anesthesiology* 51:103, 1979.
5. Holbrook PR; Mickell J; and Pollack NM: Cardiovascular Resuscitation Drugs for Children. *Crit Care Med* 8:8, 588, 762, 1980.
6. Perkin RM and Anas NG: Cardiovascular Evaluation and Support in the Critically Ill Child. *Pediatr Annals* 1986; 15:30-57.
7. Stewart RD and Lacovery DC: Administration of Endotracheal Medications. *Ann Emerg Med* 1985; 14:136.

3

ABUSE

A. Child Abuse

1. Abuse may be active (physical, sexual, psychological) or passive (physical, emotional, medical, educational neglect). Physical injury is the easiest to discern; psychological injury is the hardest.
2. If there is suspicion that a child has been abused, health care providers are legally required to report it to the proper authorities (usually Social Services). Remember, an abused child is being reported to safeguard him from further harm.
3. Always supplement medical input with input from social work, when available. Social workers have expertise in interviewing skills, which permit them to discover information that might otherwise remain hidden.
4. Approach the parent in a nonjudgmental fashion. Ask open, not leading, questions. Do not demonstrate personal prejudices, anger, or disgust. Be as compassionate as possible.
5. If the child is presenting with an injury, determine whether the story of the injury's causation fits the child's physical condition.
   a. Was there a delay in seeking medical therapy? Why?

b. Who was supervising the child at the time of the injury?

c. Has the child sustained burns, lacerations, head trauma, or fractures in the past? If yes, when and what caused these injuries?

6. Determine the child's health status and the family's living conditions.

   a. Where does he receive his well-child care?

   b. Determine whether the child has a chronic medical condition. What is it?

   c. To what support systems does the family have access?

   d. Are the parents employed? Do they have sufficient money for food, clothing, and shelter?

   e. How many persons live with the child?

   f. How many siblings does he have, what are their ages, and do they live with him?

7. Determine the child's psychosocial milieu.

   a. Was the child planned?

   b. What is his best characteristic? His worst characteristic?

   c. Who are his usual caregivers?

   d. What does he do that merits discipline? How is he usually disciplined?

   e. Does domestic violence occur? Against whom?

   f. Do any family members have difficulty with alcohol or drug abuse? Who?

   g. For children older than 2 yr: Is he toilet-trained? If yes, does he ever have accidents? If yes, how is he treated after such episodes? (N.B., Many children are abused in conjunction with toilet-training, incontinence, meal battles, and sleep problems.)

8. The child's PE is performed looking for both overt and subtle signs of abuse.

   a. Is the child clean or dirty?

   b. Fearful or calm?

   c. Clingy or aggressive?

   d. Verbal or silent?

e. Will he make eye contact with his parent? With the examiner?

f. Does he want his parent to hold him or does he prefer to go to the examiner? How does the parent react to his cries or requests? (N.B., Psychologically abused children may be timid or may be aggressive: both behaviors relate to their poor self-image. Neglected children may actually prefer the examiner to their parents).

9. A <u>thorough</u> PE is performed. Particular attention should be paid to

a. Skin markings - lacerations, burns, ecchymoses, linear contusions (belts, straps), contusions with definite shapes (coat hangers, belt buckles), circular contusions on trunk or limbs (finger pressure points), bites, etc.

b. Oral trauma - torn frenulum (forced bottle feeding or pacifier), contused gums, loose teeth (blow to mouth).

c. Nasal trauma.

d. Ear trauma.

e. Eye trauma - hyphema, periorbital hematomas, hemorrhage.

f. Chest injuries.

g. Blunt abdominal trauma.

h. Genital trauma (see "sexual abuse").

i. Limb trauma - asymmetries, fractures, dislocations, inability to walk, etc.

j. Head trauma - hematomas, lacerations, deformities. Document positives and negatives.

k. Growth parameters (should plot on growth curves).

10. Laboratory tests should be dictated by history and physical findings.

a. A urinalysis is indicated if there is evidence of acute genital, abdominal, or back trauma.

b. Evidence of active bleeding, ecchymoses, or blunt abdominal trauma suggest a complete blood count (with platelets).

    c. Deformed or tender limbs, tender ribs, abdominal, head, or chest trauma dictate radiographs. Trauma surveys (to determine past or occult fractures) are useful mainly in pre-verbal children and retarded patients, and should be done in children younger than 3 years with suspected physical abuse.

11. Photographs (labeled with the date, patient's name, and the photographer's name) of suspicious skin markings should be obtained.

12. The child's disposition should be based on both medical and social concerns.

    a. Children with moderate to severe injuries, those with unstable neurological or cardiovascular exams, and those with acute psychological disturbances should be admitted.

    b. When a child is not admitted, the decision must be made as to where he may be discharged. If the suspected abuser lives with the child, the child might be sent to another relative or to foster care. If the suspected abuser does not live with the child, he might be sent home with his parent. Ultimate placement is at the discretion of the judicial system.

    c. Siblings of the abused child also should be promptly examined and removed from the home, if necessary; solicit social service and/or police assistance in this regard.

B. Sexual Abuse

1. Sexual abuse entails engaging the child in masturbation; fondling; voyeurism; pornography; oral, anal, or genital intercourse. The use of bribes, gifts, or compliments to engage a young child in sexual acts should be regarded as forced sexual abuse.

2. A social worker should always be involved at the onset. Some communities have designated Sexual Assault and Rape Centers. Patients with recent (i.e., <48 hr) rape, genital trauma, or sexual assault

should go to such centers under police escort for evaluation, if the patient is in no other medical distress. If patient is too unstable for referral, do complete evaluation and therapy at hospital of presentation.

3. Careful documentation is mandatory. This includes a detailed history of the event written as quotations of the parents or, if appropriate, in the patient's words.
   a. Who is the alleged assailant?
   b. When and where did the episode occur?
   c. Did penile penetration occur?
   d. Did other trauma occur? What was it?
   e. Who (name and relationship) is accompanying the patient presently?
   f. Obtaining an accurate history may be difficult, and disclosure might not be immediate. Children may be fearful of revealing details or name of person.

4. A complete PE is necessary with special emphasis on the oral, perineal, and anal areas (signs of old or new trauma, pharyngitis, mouth lesions, urethral or vaginal discharge, patulous anus, anal discharge or lesions, or tender rectum).
   a. Document positive findings with properly labeled photographs or drawings.
   b. Record the appearance and size of the hymenal opening in a prepubertal child (size is generally 1 mm per year of life). Do not force an examination; consider the use of sedation.
   c. Examination by a gynecologist, perhaps under sedation or anesthesia, may be necessary. (This is especially true if active bleeding is present).

5. If very recent (<72 hr) sexual abuse is suspected, obtain the following specimens when possible and place in appropriate containers. Alternatively, send patient to a sexual assault center, if available; such a center is specially equipped to collect these specimens:
   a. Hair, if any, combed from pubic area.

b. Vaginal fluid.
   Wet mount of material examined immediately for motile sperm. Slide of vaginal secretions fixed with formalin (as with Pap smear) and sent to cytopathology for sperm.

c. GC culture: Include throat or mouth and rectum, as well as cervix/vagina, and penile urethra as appropriate.

d. Chlamydial cultures of genital secretions.

e. Swab of vaginal secretions mixed with 2 cc normal saline in test tube to be sent on ice immediately to lab for acid phosphatase to test for semen. The lab also may be able to test for sperm precipitins and ABH agglutinogens. The test may only be available through police lab via a sexual assault center.

f. Scrape any areas which may represent dried semen from skin or clothing for acid phosphatase testing.

g. Blood and urine tests:
   1) STS (repeat in 4-6 wk); keep in mind that young children might remember the "blood test" most vividly, so be as gentle as possible.
   2) Toxicology screen if appropriate.
   3) Pregnancy test (can detect pregnancy as early as 9 days after fertilization), as appropriate.
   4) Urinalysis (U/A).

6. If sexual activity occurred several days or more before:

   a. Do a complete PE, plus an external genital examination with specific regard to the vaginal introitus and rectum. Diagram abnormal findings on patient's record, if appropriate.

   b. Take a GC culture from the vagina, throat, and rectum, and obtain an STS, and a specimen for chlamydia.

   c. If <u>any</u> questions, get consultation from a knowl-
      edgeable consultant.
   d. Pregnancy test, if appropriate.
   e. U/A.
7. Arrange appropriate follow-up of the child and family. A social worker can arrange shelter if needed.
8. Counsel parents not to make a bad situation worse
   by using such terms as "ruined," "violated,", or
   "dirty." The child's emotional reaction to sexual
   abuse is magnified by the imposition of adult values, which may lead to anxiety and guilt feelings.

REFERENCES

Child Abuse

1. Mundie GE: Team Management of the Maltreated Child in the Emergency Room. *Pediatr Annals* 1984; 13:771-6.
2. Ellerstein NS and Norris KJ: Value of Radiologic Skeletal Survey in Assessment of Abused Children. *Pediatr* 1984; 74:1075-78.
3. Norton LE:Child Abuse.*Clinics in Lab Med* 1983; 3:321-42.
4. Jensen AD et al: Ocular Clues to Child Abuse. *J Pediatr Ophthalmology* 1971; 8:270-3.
5. Bittner S and Newberger EH:Pediatric Understanding of Child Abuse and Neglect. *Pedatr in Rev* 1981; 2:197-207.
6. Helfer R: The Epidemiology of Child Abuse and Neglect. *Pediatr Annals* 1984; 13:745-51.
7. Woollcott P et al: Doctor Shopping with the Child as Proxy Patient: A Variant of Child Abuse. *J Pediatr* 1982; 101:297-301.

Sexual Abuse

1. Sarles R: Sexual Abuse and Rape. *Pediatr in Rev* 1982; 4:93-8.
2. Jones J: Sexual Abuse of Children. *AJDC* 1982; 136:142-6.
3. Herman-Giddens ME and Frothingham TE: Prepubertal Female Genitalia - Examination for Evidence of Sexual Abuse. *Pediatr* 1987; 80:203-8.
4. Seidel J et al: Presentation and Evaluation of Sexual Misuse in the Emergency Department. *Pediatr Emerg Care* 1986; 2:157-64.
5. Enos W et al: Forensic Evaluation of the Sexually Abused Child. *Pediatr* 1986; 78:385-98.
6. Emans SJ et al: Genital Findings in Sexually Abused, Symptomatic, and Asymptomatic Girls. *Pediatr* 1987; 79:778-85.
7. Krugman R: Recognition of Sexual Abuse in Children. *Pediatr in Rev* 1986; 8:25-30.
8. Remsza ME and Niggemann EH: Medical Evaluation of Sexually Abused Children - A Review of 311 Cases. *Pediatr* 1982; 69:8-14.

9. Blumberg M: Sexual Abuse of Children. *Pediatr Annals* 1984; 13:753-8.
10. McCauley J et al: Toluidene Blue in the Detection of Perineal Lacerations in Pediatric and Adolescent Sexual Abuse Victims. *Pediatr* 1986; 78:1039-43.
11. Spencer M and Dunklee P: Sexual Abuse of Boys. *Pediatr* 1986; 78:133-8.
12. Horowitz DA: Physical Examination of Sexually Abused Children and Adolescents. *Pediatr in Rev* 1987; 9:25-30.

4

DERMATOLOGY

A. Acne

1. Evaluation: Score comedones, papules, and pustules on scale of 1-4+ and record location.
2. Treatment
   a. Counsel that treatment will have no effect for 4-6 wk. Don't expect complete resolution.
   b. Start with 5% benzoyl peroxide qd. If tolerated, may increase to 10% benzoyl peroxide. (3% of population is allergic to benzoyl peroxide.)
   c. You may add 0.05% Retin-A cream qd. Useful combination with benzoyl peroxide. Use Retin-A at night 20 minutes after washing and benzoyl peroxide in the day. Start Retin-A qod for first week. Apply small amount of cream to whole face, not just lesions.
   d. Systemic Antibiotics
      Useful for papulopustular acne.
      Tetracycline 500 mg bid to start, gradually reduce dosage. May increase to 1.5 gm/day for short period. Erythromycin is alternate drug.
   e. Topical Antibiotics
      Solutions are available for topical use of erythromycin and clindamycin. Use with benzoyl peroxide and/or Retin-A for papulopustular

acne with insufficient inflammation to require systemic antibiotics.

f. For nodular cystic acne, if 3 months of intensive topical therapy fails, refer to a dermatologist for treatment with Accutane.

B. Atopic Dermatitis (Eczema)

1. Characterized by erythema, edema, papules, and weeping in the active phase. Scales and lichenification may develop later. Paroxysmal and severe pruritus is associated with eczema. If there is no pruritus, it's not eczema! Pyoderma is often superimposed (staph, strep).

2. Three clinical phases
   a. Phase I: Infantile eczema (2 mo - 2 yr) - face, scalp, trunk, extensor surfaces of extremities; 1/3 of these infants will progress to Phase II.
   b. Phase II:Childhood eczema (2 yr - adolescence - flexor surfaces predominantly involved (antecubital, popliteal, neck, wrists, sometimes hands and feet).
      1) Atopic feet appear in some children during this phase involving soles of feet with cracking, erythema, and pain. May be confused with tinea pedis (athlete's foot).
      2) A third of these patients will progress to adolescent eczema.
   c. Phase III: Adolescent Eczema - hands (mostly), eyelids, neck, feet, and flexor areas may be involved.

3. History of asthma and hay fever in these patients (30%) and their families (70%).

4. Common associated findings include a tendency to dry skin, keratosis pilaris (chicken skin appearance), increased palmar markings, atopic pleats, a tendency to lichenification, and ichthyosis vulgaris.

5. A few patients may have associated immunodeficiency.

6. Treatment

a. Educate family and patient that this is a chronic, recurring disorder which can't be cured but can be controlled with conscientious therapy. It usually decreases in severity (and may disappear) with age.
b. Acute phase
   1) If weeping, use wet compresses (cottoncloth) soaked in aluminum acetate solution (Burow's solution, Domeboro 1 packet per quart of cool water). Apply 10-20 minutes, 4-6 times/d x 2-3 d. May also use plain tepid water as compress.
   2) Systemic anti-staph therapy if superimposed infection is suspected. Local Rx will not work if infection is neglected.
   3) Local steroids: Frequent application of 1% hydrocortisone cream for maintenance therapy of mild dermatitis of face and intertriginous areas. May need more potent steroid (e.g., Triamcinolone 0.1% or even fluocinonide 0.05%, e.g., Lidex) 1-3 times daily x 4-5 d. <u>Do not use fluorinated steroids on face or intertriginous areas.</u>
   4) Emollients are best for dry, scaling, or fissured eruptions. Apply Eucerin, Moisturel, Aquaphor or acid mantle cream 3-4 times/d.
   5) Baths: Aveeno (oatmeal) bath. Use 1/2 cup per half tub of tepid water x 15 minutes. Hot baths and soaps are contraindicated. N.B. This is an expensive OTC preparation that prescription plans do not cover.
   6) Antipruritics: Hydroxyzine (Vistaril or Atarax) may be used hs (1-2 mg/kg).
c. Chronic Management: Goal is hydration of skin and relief of itching.
   1) Avoid irritants (wool clothing, soaps, excessive bathing, excessive sweating). Keep as much of skin covered with cotton clothing as possible.

2) Tepid "drip-dry" bath 1-2x/week, 5 min each without soaps (except in groin, anal, axillary areas).
   a) If soap <u>must</u> be used, use mild soap (e.g., Dove).
   b) Avoid Ivory, Dial, Safeguard. With skin still wet, apply lubricant (e.g., Eucerin, Nivea, Aquaphor) liberally and PRN.
      NOTE: These preparations are OTC and expensive.
3) Steroids:use small amounts frequently (3-6x/d)
   a) Use low potency (1% hydrocortisone) for chronic use because of danger of hypopigmentation and systemic absorption.
   b) Attempt to wean off steroids as soon as possible through the liberal use of lubricants several times each day.
   c) If you can justify the use of 1% hydrocortisone, pharmacist can mix a lubricant (Eucerin) 454 gm + 1% hydrocortisone 5 gm, and prescription plans will cover the cost.
4) Hydroxyzine sometimes needed for relief of itching. Make sure fingernails are cut short.
5) Follow-up
   First visit within 1 week to review therapy, then monthly visits until patient is using lubricants only, after which q3-6 mo visits should suffice.
6) Eczema may be seen in systemic disorders, e.g., Wiskott-Aldrich syndrome, histiocytosis, and phenylketonuria.

C. Contact Dermatitis

1. Acute onset of intensely pruritic papulovesicular rash in patches and/or streaks. Can be confused with insect bites, scabies, eczema.
2. May be allergic or irritant (secondary to toxic chemicals). Common etiologies include:

a. Poison ivy, oak, sumac. Usually occurs as linear streaks. Commonly on face, extremities, and scrotum.
b. Shoe-leather allergy. Occurs on sides and dorsum of feet with sparing of interdigital areas and soles. Can be confirmed by patch testing.
c. Nickel allergy. Secondary to poor quality earrings.
d. Topical medications.

3. Treatment
a. Avoid further contact with allergen.
b. 7-10 day course of topical steroid - 1% hydrocortisone ointment to face, fluorinated steroid preparation to trunk and extremities.
c. An antihistamine may be useful to control itching.
d. If lesions are on face, widespread, or accompanied by edema (especially with poison ivy), a 10-day course of oral prednisone works like magic. Start at 2 mg/kg/d (60 mg maximum) and decrease by 5 to 10 mg each day.
N.B. Poison ivy is not just a summertime problem.

D. Diaper Rash

1. Some infants have sensitive skin predisposed to diaper dermatitis; others have seborrheic or atopic dermatitis; others may have monilial rash alone or superimposed on other dermatitis.
2. General Guidelines
a. Most important therapy for any of the above: Avoid continuous moisture and excessive heat; make frequent diaper changes. Avoid plastic pants and occlusive diapers. Keep skin dry, and air-dry diaper area as much as possible.
b. Cleanse diaper area with water at each diaper change. If soap is necessary, use a mild one (Dove).

    c. Apply frequently a protective ointment with petrolatum or zinc oxide base (e.g., A & D ointment, Desitin, zinc oxide).

    d. If pyoderma develops, use wet compresses and po antibiotic strep, staph coverage. Do not use topical antibiotics - very sensitizing.

3. Primary Irritant Dermatitis:Due to prolonged contact of skin with urine and feces with their irritating chemicals and enzymes. Characterized by erythema, thickening of skin, and $\pm$ vesicles.

    a. Rx as above (general guidelines).

    b. If skin is inflamed, brief course of steroid (1% hydrocortisone) applied with each diaper change x 5-7 d. Avoid fluorinated steroids.

    c. 80% of diaper rashes lasting >4 days are colonized with <u>Candida</u>, even before classic signs of <u>Monilia</u> rash appear. Treatment includes alternating applications of Nystatin cream with 1% steroid cream or ointment each time diaper is changed.

4. <u>Monilia</u> Rash (<u>Candida albicans</u>): Fiery red, papular lesions with peripheral scaling at times. May also be pustular. Folds involved, satellite lesions present. Often difficult to find yeast on KOH. Look for thrush in mouth.

Treatment

    a. Nystatin cream. Treatment may be required for as long as 3 weeks.

    b. Oral nystatin, only if oral lesions are present.

    c. Also see "General Guidelines."

E. Erythema Multiforme

1. Clinical Features

    a. Symmetrical distribution of lesions evolving through multiple morphologic stages, erythematous macules, papules, plaques, vesicles, and target (iris) lesions. Lesions evolve over days, not hours. (Hives evolve over hours, not days, and are not symmetric in distribution.)

b. Lesions tend to occur over dorsum of hands and feet, palms and soles, and extensor surfaces of extremities - may spread to trunk. May be associated with burning and itching. (There may be shallow mucosal ulcers, lesions.)

c. Systemic manifestations involve fever, malaise, and myalgias.

d. Stevens-Johnson Syndrome (SJS) represents a severe form of EM in which there is a prodrome of fever, malaise, myalgias, headache, and diarrhea. Followed by sudden onset of high fever, toxicity, skin eruption (EM), and inflammatory bullous lesions on mucous membranes - oral mucosa, lips, bulbar conjunctiva, and ano-genital area.

2. **Etiology**

a. Infection - viral, bacterial, fungal, protozoal, mycoplasmal. Most common antecedent illness is <u>Herpes simplex</u> virus infection.

b. Reaction to drugs, foods, immunizations.

c. Connective tissue disorders.

3. **Management**

Work-up should be aimed at finding underlying cause.

Erythema Multiforme Minor - usually mild and self-limited

a. Oral antihistamines.

b. Moist compresses.

c. Colloidal baths.

Stevens -Johnson Syndrome

a. Patient should be hospitalized.

b. Hydration.

c. Moist compresses to bullae: colloidal baths.

d. For mucosal lesions - frequent mouthwashes: local application of diphenhydramine.

e. There is no good evidence that systemic corticosteroids are effective, <u>but</u> in toxic patients they are usually used.

  f. Get ophthalmology consultation; patients prone to corneal ulcers, keratitis, uveitis, panophthalmitis.

N.B. Topical acyclovir is not effective in herpes - associated EM, but long term, maintenance oral acyclovir has been effective in preventing herpes-associated EM.

F. Impetigo

1. 2 types of lesions:
   - crusty yellow scabs = strep and staph
   - bullae = staph
2. Highly contagious - check other family members and Rx PRN.
3. Treatment: Rx for strep and lesion usually resolves
   a. Benzathine penicillin IM
      600,000 u if <30 kg 1,200,000 u if >30 kg or
   b. Erythromycin 30-50 mg/kg/d po ÷ qid x 10 d
   c. For bullae, treat with erythromycin or dicloxacillin.
   d. Use pHisohex, good scrubbing of lesions, and trim nails. Topical antibiotics aid in control of lesions but won't eradicate infections.
   e. Persistent/recurrent lesions: think reinfection vs. resistant organism:
      Rx: dicloxacillin - 40 mg/kg/d po ÷ qid x 10 d.
   f. Consider topical therapy (mupirocin) for small lesions.

G. Scabies

1. Caused by arthropod <u>Sarcoptes scabiei.</u>
2. Characterized by pruritic papules, vesicles, pustules, and linear burrows. An eczematous eruption caused by hypersensitivity to the mite can be seen. Secondary infection can also occur.
3. In older children and adults, areas of involvement - webs of the fingers, axillae, flexures of the arms and wrists, beltline, and areas around the nipples, genitals, and lower buttocks. In infants - palms, soles, head, and neck.

4. Diagnostic Procedures: Scraping of a burrow or unscratched papule covered with mineral oil. Under low power, look for mites, ova, or feces. Yield with this procedure is often low, so the diagnosis is often made by the clinical appearance.
5. Treatment:Including household contacts
   a. Lindane (available as Kwell lotion) - apply from the neck down and wash off after 6-8 hours.
   b. Crotamiton 10% (Eurax) - recommended for infants and pregnant or lactating women. Apply from the neck down nightly x 2 nights and wash off 24 hours after the second application.
   c. Clothing or bed linen possibly contaminated by the patient should be machine washed.
   NOTE: Pruritus may persist for several weeks after adequate therapy. Retreatment is indicated after 1 week; appropriate even if there is clinical improvement. Additional weekly treatments warranted only if live mites demonstrated.
   d. Family members should be treated, even in the absence of signs and symptoms.

H. Seborrheic Dermatitis

1. Characterized by erythematous, dry, scaling, crusting lesions with ± greasy, yellow appearance.
   a. Occurs in areas rich in sebaceous glands (face, scalp, perineum, postauricular and intertriginous areas).
   b. Affected areas sharply demarcated from uninvolved skin. Common in infancy (appearing between 2 and 10 wk) and puberty.
   c. Associated with cradle cap.
   d. May be confused with eczema (less itching in seborrhea).
   e. Psoriasis should also be considered in differential Dx in older children.
2. Treatment
   a. 1% hydrocortisone cream for dermatitis (not cradle cap).

  b. Keep diaper area dry.

  c. For severe cradle cap, apply baby oil to scalp x 15 min, then wash with Sebulex shampoo, or Head and Shoulders.

  d. Often must treat for candida superinfection.

I. Tinea (Dermatophyte Infections)

 1. a. Essentially 3 organisms (Trichophyton, Microsporum, Epidermophyton) cause tinea infections. Therapy is the same regardless of the organism, but differs with the site and extent of infection (topical therapy for localized skin infection; systemic therapy for widespread skin infection and infection of scalp, hair, or nails).

  b. Clinical Appearance: Expanding raised margins, scaly, ± associated scalp alopecia with visible broken hair stubble.

  c. Diagnostic Procedures:

   1) Wood's lamp - see fluorescence with skin lesions of tinea versicolor and with Microsporum scalp infections. Neither skin lesion of tinea corporis nor Trichophyton scalp infections fluoresce.

   2) KOH prep of scales, nail scrapings, or epilated hairs. Look for spores or hyphae.

   3) Send culture in uncertain cases.

 2. Tinea corporis (body - "ringworm"), cruris (genitocrural area - "jock itch"), pedis (foot - "athlete's foot"): Rx:clotrimazole (Lotrimin), tid until completely clear and then 1-2 more weeks. NOTE:

  a. Erythrasma (etiology <u>Corynebacterium minutissimum</u>) commonly confused with tinea cruris.

  b. Erythrasma not as inflamed as "jock-itch" and appears as reddish-brown, scaly patches in intertriginous areas.

  c. Treat with po erythromycin 30-50 mg/kg/d x 7d. May take weeks to completely resolve.

3. Tinea capitis (scalp and hair): Rx: micronized griseofulvin 15 mg/kg/d. Severe infections (e.g., kerions) may require 20 mg/kg/d.
   a. Give with whole milk or other food containing fat to ensure optimal absorption.
   b. At <u>least</u> 4-8 wk of griseofulvin are required for extensive skin and scalp infections.
   c. Adjunct therapy includes antiseborrheic shampoo (selenium sulfide) q 2-3 d.
4. Kerion: Circumscribed erythematous, boggy, tender scalp mass that represents an immune response to the dermatophyte and may be treated with griseofulvin as above.
   a. In some instances, there may be secondary bacterial infection, and antibiotics would be required in addition.
   b. Steroids are helpful.
   c. Start prednisone at a dose of 1-2 mg/kg/d and taper over a 10-14 d course.
5. Tinea unguim (nails): the most difficult of tinea infections to treat. Rx: griseofulvin (same dose as above).
6. Tinea versicolor: technically not a dermatophytic infection. Characterized by superficial tan or hypopigmented scaly lesions - usually on neck, upper back, chest and proximal arms. Black skin may have hypopigmented lesions. Treat with selenium sulfide solution (Selsun shampoo - OTC) or Tinver Cream (prescription).
   a. Apply to skin x 15 min, let dry, wash off.
   b. Use daily x 2-3 wk.
   c. May need to use prophylactically 1-2 times monthly.

J. **Urticaria**

1. Intensely pruritic, evanescent wheal and erythema reactions.
   a. Usually circular and well-circumscribed but can be of variable size and pattern.

   b. Angioedema (giant urticaria) consists of transient localized areas of nondependent edema.
   c. Lesions may be localized or generalized – may be associated with swelling of tongue, hypopharynx, larynx.

2. **Etiology**

   Multiple causes, but often not identified:

   a. Drugs - penicillin, ASA, nonsteroidal anti-inflammatories
   b. Food - milk, peanuts, shellfish, egg white, nuts, food additives
   c. Insect bites
   d. Infection - bacterial, viral (EBV, hepatitis), fungal parasitic
   e. Physical - heat, cold, exercise
   f. Direct skin contact - medication, chemicals, animal dander

   With chronic (>6 wk) urticaria, think of lymphoma (very rare), collagen disease, psychogenic causes. Consider w/u if symptoms suggestive of systemic condition are present. May be helpful for family to keep symptom diary. Skin tests only helpful if food, food additive, or penicillin is suspected allergen.

3. **Treatment**

   a. Acute:

      1) 1:1000 epinephrine 0.01 cc/kg SQ
      2) Antihistamines
         Hydroxyzine (Atarax, Vistaril)
         (0.5 – 1.0 mg/kg/dose q 4–6h IM;
         2 mg/kg/d q 6h po
         Cyproheptadine (Periactin) 2-4 mg q 8 - 12 h
         Diphenhydramine (Benadryl)
         12.5 mg/kg q 4-6h
      3) If severe, short course of po prednisone.
      4) Topical steroids of <u>no</u> benefit.

   N.B. Patients with recurrent acute episodes should keep an EpiPen kit (0.15 or 0.30 mg epinephrine self-injector) handy.

    b. Chronic:
       1) Try to identify and avoid allergen - possible in only 20-30% of cases.
       2) Antihistamines may be helpful.
       3) Steroids not usually indicated.

K. Viral Rashes

1. Gianotti-Crosti Syndrome (Papular Acrodermatitis of Childhood)
   a. Multiple non-pruritic, 5-10 mm, pink-red papules over face, arms, legs, buttocks, palms, and soles. The lesions fade slowly over 4-10 weeks with mild desquamation. There may be generalized lymphadenopathy and mild hepatomegaly.
   b. In some parts of the world (not U.S.) may be associated with hepatitis B infection.
   c. No treatment is required.
2. Herpes Simplex
   a. Cold Sores
      Grouped vesicles on an erythematous base. Most common on the mucocutaneous border of the lips, but may occur anywhere on the body.
   b. Primary Gingivostomatitis
      Small vesicles on the gingiva, tongue, buccal mucosa, and lips. After the vesicle breaks, a ragged shallow ulcer with an erythematous base remains - often covered by a yellowish crust. Episodes are often accompanied by fever and irritability and may last 7-10 d.
   c. Treatment is symptomatic
      1) 1/2 strength peroxide mouthwash.
      2) Cold, non-acidic fluids
      3) Viscous Xylocaine should be avoided
   d. Herpetic Whitlow
      Painful bullous crusted lesions of the fingers. Often confused with paronychia. Common in medical personnel. May spread following inappropriate I + D. Often recurrent.

N.B. Herpes genital infections are uncommon in prepubertal children and should always raise suspicion of sexual abuse.

L. Warts

1. Common Warts
   Usually found on dorsum of hands and fingers. Treatment regimens include:
   a. Benign neglect - most will involute over a 2 yr period.
   b. Keratolytics (Duofilm - lactic acid and salicylic acid in flexible collodion) - apply each evening-soak for 5 minutes before application – cover with adhesive tape – remove in morning. Reapply Duofilm next evening – continue until wart clears.
   c. If Duofilm unsuccessful - refer to dermatologist for "cccc Rx" - cutting, cautery, chemical, or cold (liquid nitrogen).
   d. Rub wart with potato cut in half, and throw over the right shoulder in the lee of a tree; bury where it lands (Tunnessen). This has to be done at midnight in the light of a full moon!

2. Subungual and Periungual Warts
   These are a real challenge!
   Treament
   a. Apply cantharidin (cantharone) in collodion over surface of wart and occlude for 24 hr. May repeat treatment in 2-3 wk.
   b. Wrap involved finger with common adhesive tape - first longitudinally and then circumferentially. Tape is removed for 12 hours every 6 1/2 d and then reapplied. This sounds like voodoo but often works after 3-4 wk.
   c. If "a" and "b" do not work, refer to dermatologist for "cccc Rx" outlined above.

3. Plantar Warts
   Treatment
   a. Pare away superficial thickened skin over the wart - apply a piece of 40% salicylic acid plaster - cover with tape. Remove the acid plaster every 2-3 d - pare the area - reapply plaster. Repeat until wart has cleared.
   b. If "a" is unsuccessful, refer to dermatologist.

REFERENCES

Acne
1. Lucky AW: Update on acne vulgaris. *Pediatr Annals* 1987; 16:29-38.
2. Shalitaar, Smith EB, Baver E: Topical erythromycin vs. clindamycin therapy for acne: Multicenter, double-blind comparison. *Arch Dermatol* 1984; 120:351.
3. Strauss JS, Rapini RP, Shalita AR, et al: Isotretinoin therapy for acne: Results of a multicenter dose-response study. *J Am Acad Dermat* 1984; 10:490.

Atopic Dermatitis
1. Hanifen JM: Atopic dermatitis. *J Am Acad Dermat* 1981; 6:113.
2. Fritz KA, Weston WL: Topical glucocorticosteroids. *Ann Allergy* 1983; 50:68-76.
3. Hurwitz S: Eczematous eruptions in childhood. *Pediatr in Rev* 3 1981; 3:23.
4. Krowchuk D: Practical aspects of the diagnosis and management of atopic dermatitis. *Pediatr Annnals* 1987; 16:57-66.
5. Sampson HA, McCaskell CC: Food hypersensitivity and atopic dermatitis. *J Pediatr* 107;669-675.

Contact Dermatitis
1. Tunnessen WW Jr: Poison ivy, oak and sumac: The three witches of summer. *Contemp Pediatr* 1985; 2:24.

Diaper Rash
1. Jacobs AH: Eruptions in the diaper area. *Ped Clin N Amer* 1978; 25:209-224.
2. Weston WL, Lane AT, Weston JA: Diaper dermatitis: Current concepts. *Pediatr* 1980; 66:532-536.

Erythema Multiforme
1. Lemake MA, Duvic M, Bean SF: Oral acyclovir for the prevention of herpes-associated erythema multiforme. *J Am Acad Dermatol* 1986; 15:50-54.
2. Ting HC, Adam BA. Erythema multiforme - response to corticosteroid. *Dermatologica* 1984; 169:175-178.

Impetigo
1. Lookingbill DP: Impetigo. *Pediatr in Rev* 1985; 7:177-181.
Scabies
1. Hurwitz S: Scabies. *Pediatr Annals* 1980; 11:226.
2. Lane AT: Scabies and head lice. *Pediatr Annals* 1987; 16:51-54.
Seborrheic Dermatitis
1. Allen HB, Honig PJ: Scaling scalp diseases in children. *Clin Pediatr* 1983; 22:
2. Williams ML: Differential diagnosis of seborrheic dermatitis. *Pediatr in Rev* 1986; 7:204-211.
Tinea
1. Ginsburg CM, McCracken GH Jr, Petruska M: Effect of feeding on bioavailability of griseofulvin in children. *J Pediatr* 1983; 102:309-311.
2. Frieden IJ: Diagnosis and management of tinea capitis. *Pediatr Annals* 1987; 16:39-48.
3. Krowchuk DP, Lucky W, Primner SI, et al: Current status of the identification and management of tinea capitis. *Pediatr* 1983; 72:625-631.
4. Tanz RR, et al: Ketoconazole vs griseofulvin for tinea capitis. *J Pediatr* 1988; 112:987.
Viral Rashes
1. Spear KL, Winkelman RK: Gianotti-Crosti syndrome: A review of ten cases not associated with hepatitis B. *Arch Dermat* 1984; 120:891-896.
Warts
1. Bunney MH, Nolan MW, Williams DA: An assessment of treating viral warts by comparative treatment trials based on a standard design. *Br J Dermat* 1976; 94:667-679.
2. Gellis SS: Warts and molluscum contagiosum in children. *Pediatr Annals* 1987; 16:69-76.

5

ENDOCRINOLOGY

A. Diabetes

1. Diabetes mellitus is a chronic metabolic disorder in which there is hyperglycemia, generally secondary to insulin lack or, less commonly, antagonism.
   a. There are two major types of primary diabetes – insulin-dependent (type I, IDDM) and non-insulin dependent (type II, NIDDM).
   b. In IDDM, the insulin-producing capacity of the pancreas is severely limited due to loss of beta cell function.
   c. In NIDDM, which occurs occasionally in children, there is often insulin resistance due to obesity or insulin receptor abnormalities.
2. Secondary diabetes may occur when there is insulin antagonisim (excess glucocorticoid, hyperthyroidism, pheochromocytoma, growth hormone excess), unavailable glucose (glycogen storage disease), or with the use of certain drugs (thiazide diuretics).
3. Important historical information includes weight loss, polydypsia, polyphagia, polyuria (especially nocturia or nocturnal enuresis),general health, moods, school performance, and a family history of diabetes.

4. Unless there has been weight loss or there is marked obesity (NIDDM), the physical exam is usually normal; the exception is the patient in diabetic ketoacidosis (see next section).

5. Laboratory tests include assessment of fasting blood glucose concentrations (suggestive: Fasting level >120 mg/dl) or 2-hour post prandial glucose concentrations (>180 mg/dl) on two separate occasions. If elevated glucose concentrations are discovered coincidentally during a well child or acute illness visit, a glucose tolerance test should be done. The child is given 1.75 g/kg (maximum 100g) of glucose in an oral solution. Both insulin and glucose concentrations are measured at the onset and at 30, 60, 90, 120, 180, and 240 minutes.

6. Treatment
   a. Insulin - The new diabetic usually requires 0.5 - 1.0 u/kg/d of insulin, but this depends on the child's stage of puberty.
      1) If control can be achieved in a single daily injection, one-half to two-thirds of the dose is an intermediate-acting insulin (NPH or lente), and one-third is rapid-acting (regular insulin).
      2) Both types are drawn into the same syringe and injected SQ just before breakfast if single daily injection.
      3) If hyperglycemia is present between breakfast and lunch, the amount of regular insulin may be increased; if hyperglycemia is present later in the day, the amount of intermediate insulin may be increased.
      4) If two daily doses of insulin are needed, about two-thirds of the daily dose is usually given in the morning and one-third in the late afternoon before dinner.
      5) The proportion of intermediate to rapid insulin in each injection is usually about 2-3:1.
      6) Increases or decreases should be on the order of 10% at a time.

7) Blood glucose concentrations and ketonuria are assessed before meals and at bedtime.

8) In times of medical, surgical, or emotional stress, additional insulin may be needed.

b. Diet - The diabetic child requires the proper calories and nutrients to control his disease and promote adequate growth.

1) Prior to puberty, total intake usually approximates 1000 calories plus 100 calories/yr of life.

2) The diet should be composed of roughly 55% carbohydrates (starches rather than simple sugar), 30% fat (polyunsaturated, vegetable sources), and 15% protein.

3) Twenty percent of the calories should be consumed at breakfast, 20% at lunch, 30% at dinner, and 30% divided into three snacks, but this is dependent on each individual's activity level. Meals should be timed on a regular basis.

c. Exercise - The child with diabetes needs adequate exercise. He should always have a simple sugar with him in case he becomes hypoglycemic during exercise. If this occurs repeatedly, his diet should be adjusted or his insulin dosage should be decreased by 10%.

d. Hypoglycemia - The symptoms of hypoglycemia are due to catecholamine release (trembling, sweating, tachycardia) and to cerebral glucopenia (sleepiness, confusion, mood changes, seizures, coma).

1) Causes include excess insulin, decreased oral intake, and exercise without a concomitant increase in calories.

2) The diabetic child and his family should be educated in depth about these episodes. If alert, the hypoglycemic child may ingest a carbohydrate snack to abort the attack. Monogel Instant Glucose or cake icing can be ap-

plied to the buccal mucosa in children who are vomiting.

3) The child who is seizing, stuporous, or vomiting intractably should receive intravenous glucose and/or 0.5 mg glucagon IM.

e. Psychological support for both patient and parents.

f. The diabetic child should be managed in conjunction with an endocrinologist.

B. Diabetic Ketoacidosis (DKA)

1. DKA is a state of metabolic derangement in which the patient is acidotic, has an elevated serum glucose, and has serum ketones present; the acidosis is secondary to the ketosis. DKA occurs at times of physical or emotional stress, infectious illness, and noncompliance with insulin therapy. Frequently, new diabetics present in DKA.

2. Important historical information includes whether the patient is a known diabetic, his usual (and last) insulin dose, his diet in the previous 24 hours, and whether he is ill (and the symptoms thereof) or stressed, physically or emotionally.

3. The PE of the patient in DKA frequently reveals him to be weak, sleepy, lethargic or frankly comatose. He might be dehydrated (severely). If he is awake, he might complain of abdominal pain, nausea, or vomiting. He might have a fruity odor (ketosis) to his breath and demonstrate Kussmaul respirations.

4. In a patient in whom DKA is suspected, the following baseline studies should be done stat:

a. Dextrostix/chemstrip	- glucose
b. Serum acetone	- positive
c. Serum glucose	- elevated
d. Venous pH	- low
e. Serum CO_2	- low
f. Serum BUN	- normal, or high
g. Serum PO_4	- low

    h. Serum K   - low, normal or high
    i. Serum Ca   - low - normal
    j. Urine glucose/ketones   - elevated

5. The patient in DKA constitutes a medical emergency. Begin treatment immediately.
   a. Fluids
      1) Assess hydration (The patient with DKA will be dry.)
      2) Administer normal saline at 20 cc/kg/h x 1-2 hr.
      3) Then, administer half normal saline to replace deficit plus maintenance and ongoing losses over 24 hr.
   b. Insulin
      1) Administer 0.1 u regular insulin/kg by IV bolus.
      2) Follow with insulin drip of 0.1 u regular insulin/kg/h. piggybacked into IV line (i.e., 50 u insulin per 250 cc saline). An insulin drip is preferable to repeated boluses to maintain finer control of the serum glucose.

         A fresh insulin solution should be made every 16h, at least, and is preferably administered through an IMED. Never delay starting an insulin drip because the patient already had his dose of insulin.
   c. Glucose
      1) Measure detrostix/chemstrip qh.
      2) Measure serum glucose q 3-4 h (more frequently early in therapy).
      3) Rate of glucose fall should be 80-100 mg/dl/h.
         a) If glucose falls <50 mg/dl/h, increase insulin rate.
         b) If glucose falls >100 mg/dl/h, continue insulin drip (0.1 u/kg/h) and add D_5W to IV.
      4) When serum glucose approaches 250-300 mg/dl, add D_5W to IV, even if this is early in therapy.

5) When serum glucose is <200-250 mg/dl, and if ketonemia is still present, decrease insulin drip/rate to 0.05 u/kg/h.

d. Acidosis

1) Administer bicarbonate <u>only if</u> pH <7.10, serum HCO_5 <5; the dose is 2 mEq/kg $NaHCO_3$ IV over 30-60 minutes <u>or</u> added to the first bottle of half-normal saline.

2) Follow venous pH and HCO_3- q 2-4 h.

e. Serum ketones

1) Initially measure with serum glucose.

2) B-hydroxybutyrate is not measured by acetest tablets; but as therapy progresses, it converts to a measurable ketone, acetoacetate. This can give the false impression that ketosis is worsening.

f. Electrolytes

1) Follow serum electrolytes q 3-4 hr.

2) Phosphate

a) Depleted in DKA.

b) Will be further depleted with therapy.

c) Replace with potassium phosphate (see potassium below).

3) Potassium

a) Depleted in DKA, even though serum K can be "normal," high, or low.

b) ECG can be used to follow K.

c) Withhold K at the beginning of therapy if serum K is elevated or patient is anuric.

d) Administer maintenance plus deficit K over 24 hr. Replace K, half as KCl and half as potassium phosphate for first 8 hours, <u>then</u> as all KCl. A general guide is that you can give 40 meq/liter if initial K is less than normal. In severe hypokalemia, large K inputs are necessary. Patients must have cardiac monitoring while receiving K.

g. Monitor vital signs, fluid intake and output.

C. Hypoglycemia

1. Hypoglycemia is defined as a low serum glucose concentration: (premature infant< 20 mg/dl; term infant 1-3 days old < 30 mg/dl; infant < 40 mg/dl; children < 50 mg/dl).
   a. Hypoglycemia may result from prolonged or excessive insulin secretion or from disturbances in gluconeogenesis or glycogenolysis, as occurs when there are excessive body needs (e.g., sick premies).
2. Symptoms of hypoglycemia are due to epinephrine secretion (tachycardia, diaphoresis, flushing, anxiety, weakness, hunger) and to cerebral glucopenia (confusion, behavior changes, stupor, seizures, coma).
   a. If severe and prolonged, hypoglycemia may cause brain damage.
   b. In the neonate, hypoglycemia symptoms include jitteriness, pallor, diaphoresis, hypothermia, weakness, difficulty feeding, apathy, seizures, apnea/tachypnea.
3. Important historical information includes the presence of the aforementioned symptoms and their timing and frequency, the possibility of drug or toxin ingestion, the patient's growth and general health, and a family history of similar episodes.
4. The physical exam should be complete.
5. Causes of hypoglycemia
   a. Neonatal hypoglycemia (secondary to hepatic enzyme immaturity, reduced hepatic glycogen stores due to in utero malnutrition, sepsis, severe systemic illness, hyperinsulinism due to maternal diabetes or hyperplasia (nesidioblastosis) of beta cells or islets).
   b. Postprandial (postprandial hypersecretion of insulin or heightened tissue response to normal insulin levels). Leucine-associated hypoglycemia (usually familial) occurs because leucine stimulates insulin secretion; afflicted patients have increased numbers of beta cells.

c. Fasting (hyperinsulinism).

d. Deficiency of hormones regulating serum glucose levels (growth hormone, ACTH, catecholamines, thyroid hormone, cortisol, glucagon).

e. Defective liver enzymes which control gluconeogenesis/glycogenolysis (glycogen storage disease, galactosemia, maple syrup urine disease, fructose metabolism disorders).

f. Adrenal Disease (insufficiency, congenital adrenal hypoplasia).

g. Hepatic Disease (insults due to tumors, leukemia, hepatitis, toxins).

h. Ketotic Hypoglycemia: Common form of hypoglycemia in children. It is thought to be secondary to endogenous gluconeogenic amino acids (notably alanine). Attacks occur in the morning, are associated with stress, fasting, or infection, and respond rapidly to glucose administration. Such children are normal between attacks.

i. Early stages of NIDDM (erratic insulin secretion), exercise-induced hypoglycemia in diabetes, insulin overdose.

j. Miscellaneous (drugs-insulin, alcohol, salicylates, propranolol; kwashiorkor; Reye's syndrome).

6. Laboratory tests are dictated by the findings of the history and physical exam. A 5-hr glucose tolerance test may be useful. Other tolerance tests include glucagon (challenges the liver's glycogenolysis potential) and alanine (challenges the liver's gluconeogenesis potential). The workups of hyperinsulinism and hormonal deficiencies are very important.

7. Acute treatment of hypoglycemia includes glucose administration orally or intravenously.

a. If the child is alert, he should be encouraged to drink carbohydrate solutions; if he is incapable of taking oral fluids, he should receive intravenous glucose (10-25% dextrose solution).

b. Glucagon (0.5 mg IM) may also terminate the attack, but is useful only in hyperinsulinemic children. Blood glucose and insulin levels should be followed.

Long-term management is tailored to the underlying disorder causing the attacks. Children with ketotic hypoglycemia should be fed frequently; those with hormonal deficiencies may respond to their exogenous replacement; those with enzyme deficiencies should receive the appropriate diet; and those with hyperinsulinism may improve with diazoxide (10 mg/kg/d divided bid).

8. Both patient and parents require psychological support.

9. The hypoglycemic patient should be managed in conjunction with an endocrinologist.

D. Hyperthyroidism

1. Hyperthyroidism results from excessive secretion of thyroid hormone.

a. There is a neonatal variant (usually 2° to maternal hyperthyroidism) and the more common acquired type. A diffuse goiter is generally present. Hyperthyroidism is usually considered to be a manifestation of an autoimmune disease.

b. The sex ratio is equal in the congenital variant; in the acquired variant, the female to male ratio is 5:1.

2. Important historical information includes the child's appetite (usually voracious with little or no weight gain or weight loss); mental state (restless, irritable, hyperactive, anxious); presence of tremors; exophthalmos (uncommon in children); excessive sweating; and increased stool frequency. The older patient may complain of palpitations.

3. The PE should be complete with particular attention to vital signs (elevated heart rate and widened pulse pressure), ocular exam (exophthalmos), cardiac assessment (decompensation may occur, especially in infants), and the thyroid exam (size, appearance, consistency, presence of a bruit).
   a. In thyroid "storm" (malignant hyperthyroidism, which is rare in pediatrics), the patient may present with hyperthermia, tachycardia, delirium, or coma; such a "storm" may be fatal.
4. Laboratory tests include measurement of thyroxine (T_4) and triiodothyronine (T_3) by RIA; both are elevated as is the T_3 resin uptake. Long-acting thyroid stimulator (LATS) is found in 50% of patients. Antithyroglobulin antibodies may be present.
5. Treatment modalities include surgical and medical approaches, but surgery is usually performed <u>only</u> if medical therapy is unsuccessful or not feasible.
   a. Medical therapy of congenital hyperthyroidism consists of Lugol's solution (1 gtt q 8 h) and propylthiouracil (5-7 mg/kg/d ÷ q8h).
   b. If the infant is ill (especially cardiac decompensation), parenteral fluids, digoxin, and propranolol may be necessary.
   c. Medical therapy of acquired hyperthyroidism consists of propylthiouracil (5-7 mg/kg/d ÷ q8h) or methimazole (0.4-0.7 mg/kg/d ÷ q8h); drug dosage is carefully titrated to the child's response, since excess medication can precipitate hypothyroidism. Treatment continues for at least 2 yr and should be tapered slowly before complete discontinuation.
   d. The hyperthryoid patient should be managed in conjunction with an endocrinologist.

E. **Hypothyroidism**

1. Hypothyroidism results from deficient production of thyroid hormones. There is a congenital variant and an acquired type.

2. In the congenital form (cretinism), early (first weeks of life) signs/symptoms include prolonged neonatal jaundice, poor appetite and suck (large tongue), choking and/or dyspnea with feeding, constipation, infrequent cry, sluggishness, hypothermia, and bradycardia.

   a. If such a patient's condition remains uncorrected for the first 3-6 mo of life, he will likely display growth retardation, large fontanelles, hypertelorism with periorbital puffiness, a flat nose, a gaping mouth with a protruding enlarged tongue, hoarse cry, short neck, sparse hair, hypotonicity, and apathy.

   b. If he remains untreated, both physical and mental development will be retarded.

3. In the acquired form, the patient may have apathy, dry skin, hypothermia, and constipation.

   a. Depending on age and duration of symptoms, physical growth and development may be affected to a greater or lesser degree.

   b. The thyroid gland may be enlarged or small.

   c. In lymphocytic thyroiditis, the gland is nodular, firm, and nontender; in suppurative thyroiditis, which is a rare cause of hypothyroidism, the gland is tender, large, and warm with redness of the overlaying skin.

4. Causes of hypothyroidism

   a. <u>Pituitary disease</u> (global).

   b. <u>Deficiency of thyroid-stimulating hormone (TSH)</u> or <u>thyroid-releasing hormone (TRH).</u>

   c. <u>Thyroid gland dysgenesis</u> (absence, hypoplasia, ectopia).

   d. <u>Thyroid gland dysfunction/enzyme deficiencies</u> (defects in iodide trapping, oxidation or incorporation into hormones, defects in thyroglobulin synthesis, hormone production , storage, or release).

   e. <u>Suppurative thyroiditis</u> ($2°$ to infection or trauma); rare cause of hypothyroidism.

    f. <u>Autoimmune thyroiditis (Hashimoto's disease):</u> Most common form of acquired hypothyroidism with female to male ratio 4-7:1. Gland is infiltrated by lymphocytes and plasma cells. At least half of affected patients have antithyroid antibodies. Familial clustering occurs. It is associated with other autoimmune diseases, Down's and Turner's syndromes.

    g. <u>Lack of dietary iodine</u> (rare).

    h. <u>S/P subtotal thyroidectomy.</u>

    i. <u>Antihyperthyroid medication overdose.</u>

    j. <u>Maternal ingestion of iodides or antihyperthyroid medications during pregnancy.</u>

5. Historical information and PE should elicit signs and symptoms as listed in numbers 2 and 3 above.

6. Laboratory tests include measurement of T_3 and T_4 (low or borderline), T_3 resin uptake (low), and TSH (high if defect in thyroid, low if defect in pituitary or hypothalamus).

    a. If TSH is low, administration of TRH will assist in determining if defect is in the pituitary or hypothalamus (TSH rise with TRH administration signifies TRH deficiency and a hypothalamic defect; TSH unchanged with TRH implies pituitary failure).

7. a. Neonatal screening identifies the majority of patients with congenital hypothyroidism.

    b. Treatment of congenital hypothyroidism must be prompt if growth retardation and mental retardation are to be avoided.

    c. Since a good portion of T_3 is derived from T_4, the hypothyroid patient may be treated with oral sodium-L-thyroxine (newborn infants: initially $10\mu g/kg/d$); older children and adolescents: $100\text{-}250\mu g/d$).

    d. The patient with suppurative thyroiditis merits incision and drainage of the gland with appropriate antibiotic therapy.

e. Patients with hypothyroidism should be managed in conjunction with an endocrinologist.

F. **Short Stature**

1. In infants, short stature may be associated with overall failure to thrive. In older children and adolescents, short stature may be an isolated finding.
2. Short stature may be due to growth failure or to marked deceleration of growth, so that the individual "falls from" his prior height percentile.
3. Important historical information includes prenatal and birth histories, pattern of growth, presence of chronic disease, chronic medication use, developmental milestones, and the growth and pubertal pattern of parents and siblings.
4. A thorough PE is mandatory; however, most individuals with short stature have normal exams.
5. The causes of short stature are numerous.
   a. Genetic or familial (heights of relatives will be useful).
   b. Constitutional delay: Normal growth in early infancy with deceleration of growth by late infancy, early toddlerhood, or early childhood years. Puberty, height, and bone age are delayed by 2-4 years; however, adult height is usually normal.
   c. Small-for-gestational age.
   d. Malnutrition or malabsorption (lack of calories for growth).
   e. Chronic debilitating disease, especially inflammatory bowel disease (depletion of calories).
   f. Emotional deprivation (? hypothalamic suppression).
   g. Medications (steroids, ritalin, dexedrine).
   h. Endogenous cortisol excess (Cushing's syndrome): Other associated signs are moon facies, hirsutism, buffalo hump, striae, hypertension, fatigue, deepening of the voice, obesity, and amenorrhea.

      i. Cartilage or skeletal dysplasia (short extremities with normal-sized head and trunk).

      j. Turner's syndrome (genotype 45 XO and related forms): Other associated signs are webbed neck, small jaw, prominent ears, epicanthal folds, low posterior hairline, a broad chest, and cardiac defects.

      k. Pituitary dysgenesis/dysfunction: Growth may be normal initially, but usually by age 1-2 yrs, growth is retarded and the body habitus is infantile. Other signs of pituitary dysfunction may be evident.

      l. Hypothyroidism

      m. Miscellaneous - Hypoparathyroidism and rickets.

6. Laboratory tests are dictated by the history and PE. Bone age should be assessed.

7. a. Treatment includes reassurance in most cases; provision of adequate calories for growth and proper control of chronic illnesses are mandatory.

      b. Use of growth hormone and/or thyroid hormone in appropriate individuals.

      c. Management of the child with short stature may be facilitated by consultation with an endocrinologist.

G. Gynecomastia

1. Gynecomastia in the adolescent male means unilateral or bilateral breast enlargement usually due to transient estrogen/testosterone imbalance.

      a. It usually begins at Tanner stage II-III, lasts for several mo, and gradually disappears within 1-2 yr.

      b. The most common finding is a small, tender, oval subareolar mass measuring up to 2-3 cm in diameter. The mass is not fixed and there is no overlying skin dimpling.

       c. Massive gynecomastia may indicate a major endocrine abnormality, perhaps in assocation with other abnormalities of sexual maturation.

  2. Important historical information includes the duration of breast enlargement, breast symptoms, and pubertal progression.

  3. A complete PE usually reveals only the breast enlargement with the remainder of the exam being normal. However, the testes must be palpated as gynecomastia may be the first sign of tumor.

  4. Common causes of gynecomastia
      a. Normal variant (adolescent gynecomastia).
      b. Pseudogynecomastia (due to obesity or increased muscle mass).
      c. Klinefelter's syndrome (47 XXY).
      d. Drug use (estrogens, chorionic gonadotropins, steroids, tricyclic antidepressants, methadone, marijuana, amphetamines, digitalis, cimetidine).
      e. Testicular tumor, liver cancer.

  5. Treatment consists of reassurance of the patient in most cases; discontinuation of offending medications may help. Massive gynecomastia requires surgical correction.

H. Premature Thelarche

  1. Premature thelarche is breast development without other signs of puberty. It may be due to exogenous estrogen (not "true" precocious thelarche) or due to slight increase in endogenous estrogen release.

  2. The condition usually appears in girls 1-4 yr of age. Breast buds of 2-4 cm are evident without nipple or areola involvement. The child may complain of breast tenderness and one breast may be more involved than the other. No growth acceleration is noted.

3. Important historical information includes growth pattern and use of medications or creams containing estrogen.

4. The PE should be complete. Note the appearance and size of the breasts. Note also the appearance of the vaginal mucosa. A rectal exam should be done to detect ovarian and uterine enlargement.

5. a. Laboratory tests <u>may</u> include a bone age assessment (normal in premature thelarche), a skull film (to rule out a process in the sella), a vaginal smear for estrogen effect, and a pelvic ultrasound (to rule out organ enlargement or masses).

   b. In many cases, no laboratory tests are indicated.

   c. If premature puberty is suspected, CNS imaging is preferable to skull films.

6. Treatment consists of close follow-up to detect other signs of puberty, discontinuation of estrogen preparations, and reassurance. Breast development frequently regresses. The onset of puberty usually occurs at the normal age. Follow-up is extremely important.

I. Premature Adrenarche

1. Premature adrenarche is the appearance of pubic hair (with or without axillary hair) before age 8 yr without estrogen effects or other androgenic signs.

2. The condition is probably due to increased hormonal production by the adrenal gland, as urinary 17-keto-steroids are generally slightly elevated for the patient's age.

3. Important historical information includes that obtained for precocious puberty (see next section).

4. A complete PE is mandatory, including a careful genital exam. Breast enlargement is usually absent; no estrogen effects are evident. Virilization is absent. The growth velocity and clitoral size must be evaluated.

5. Laboratory tests include bone age assessment (us-

ually normal or only slightly advanced), vaginal smear (should be prepubertal pattern, indicated if estrogen effect also prominent), a 24 h urine for 17-ketosteroids, and serum androgens.

6. The patient and the family should be reassured; she should be carefully followed to note any progression of development, especially height or bone age acceleration. If virilization occurs, an ovarian or adrenal tumor or adrenal hypersecretion should be suspected.

J. Precocious Puberty

1. Precocious Puberty is present when pubertal development begins before age 8 in girls and age 9 in boys.
   a. Isosexual precocious puberty refers to development appropriate to one's own sex, while heterosexual precocity refers to development appropriate to the opposite sex.

2. Important historical information includes:
   a. Prenatal and birth histories.
   b. Age of attainment of developmental milestones.
   c. Growth pattern.
   d. The presence of chronic medical conditions or chronic use of medications.
   e. A past history of encephalitis, seizures, head trauma, hydrocephalus, headaches, visual symptoms, behavior changes, abdominal pain, and genitourinary symptoms.
   f. A family history of neurofibromatosis, tuberous sclerosis, and McCune-Albright syndrome.
   g. If the patient is a boy, information on the ages of pubertal attainment of the father and brothers is necessary.
   h. If the patient is a girl, the ages of menarche of sisters, mother, and grandmothers should be elicited.

3. The PE must be complete. Emphasis should be placed on the neurological exam, the ophthalmo-

logic evaluation (fundoscopic and visual fields assessment), and the genital exam (Tanner staging of pubic hair, genitalia, and breasts). A rectal exam should be performed in girls to exclude the possibility of an ovarian mass.

4. Causes of precocious puberty
   a. Idiopathic (premature activation of hypothalamic-pituitary axis for unknown reason): 80% of girls but less than 50% of boys with premature puberty have this diagnosis.
   b. Pituitary/hypothalamic disease (post-injury, hemorrhage, tumor, hydrocephalus, post-infectious).
   c. Neurofibromatosis, tuberous sclerosis, McCune-Albright (café au lait spots, fibrous dysplasia, bone cysts).
   d. Gonadotropin-secreting tumors (teratoma, hepatoblastoma, chorioepithelioma).
   e. Ovarian tumors (granulosa cell tumor, arrhenoblastoma, lipid cell tumor, thecoma, dysgerminoma, cyst).
   f. Testicular tumors (Leydig cell tumor, seminoma).
   g. Adrenal tumor or hyperplasia.
   h. Exogenous estrogen therapy.
   i. Anabolic steroid therapy.
   j. Androgen therapy.
   k. Hypothyroidism.
5. Initial laboratory tests include a
   a. CT scan (to determine presence of an intracranial lesion in the hypothalamus).
   b. Bone age assessment (advanced in precocious puberty; delayed in hypothyroidism).
   c. Serum FSH and LH levels (high LH level suggests gonadotropin-secreting tumor or choriocarcinoma).
   d. Thyroid function tests, 24-h urine for 17-ketosteroids (if androgenization is present).
6. If an ovarian tumor is suspected by physical exam, an abdominal ultrasound or CT scan should be

obtained.

a. Depending on the type of ovarian tumor, various hormones will be elevated in the serum (estradiol with granulosa cell tumors; progesterone with thecomas).

b. A vaginal smear to determine the amount of estrogen or progesterone effect may be useful.

7. If adrenal pathology is suspected (i.e., heterosexual precocious puberty in a girl), an abdominal CT scan is useful.

a. In addition to a 24-h urine for 17-ketosteroids and pregnanetriol, a serum testosterone level should be obtained.

b. If urine 17-ketosteroids are normal and serum testosterone level is elevated, an ovarian tumor is likely.

c. If there is an elevated 17-ketosteroids level that is suppressible by dexamethasone, congenital adrenal hyperplasia is likely; if the level is not suppressible, an adrenal or gonadal tumor is likely. Dexamethasone suppression should be performed by an endocrinologist.

8. a. The first rule of treatment is to reassure and support the child. Parents should be encouraged to treat their child in an age-appropriate fashion.

b. Tumors should be removed, if possible.

c. Congenital adrenal hyperplasia is treated with glucocorticoid therapy.

d. Idiopathic and several variants of central precocious puberty in girls may be treated (only under an endocrinologist's direction) with an LHRH analog.

References

Diabetes
1. Golden M, et al: Management of diabetes mellitus in children younger than 5 years of age. *AJDC* 1985; 139:448-52.
2. Tamborlane WV, Sherwin RS: Diabetes control and complications - New strategies and insights. *J Pediatr* 1983; 102:805-13.
3. Reynolds J: Nutritional management of children and adolescents with insulin-dependent diabetes mellitus. *Pediatr in Rev* 1987; 9:155-672.
4. Schiffrin A: Management of childhood diabetes. *Pediatr Annals* 1987; 16:694-710.
5. Chase HP: Avoiding the short and long-term complications of juvenile diabetes. *Pediatr in Rev* 1985; 7:140-9.
6. Skyler JS, Rabinovitch A: Etiology and pathogenesis of insulin-dependent diabetes mellitus. *Pediatr Annals* 1987; 16:682-92.

DKA
1. Kreisberg RA: Diabetic ketoacidosis: New concepts and trends in pathogenesis and treatment. *Ann Int Med* 1978; 88:681-95.
2. Lightner ET, et al: Low-dose intravenous insulin infusion in patients with diabetic ketoacidosis - Biochemical effects in children. *Pediatr* 1977; 60:681-8.
3. Schiffer A: Management of childhood diabetes. *Pediatr Annals* 1987; 16:694-710.

Hypoglycemia
1. Cornblath M: Hypoglycemia in infancy and childhood. *Pediatr Annals* 1981; 10:356-63.
2. Pagliara A, et al: Hypoglycemia in infancy and childhood I. *Pediatr* 1973; 82:365-79.
3. Pagliara A, et al: Hypoglycemia in infancy and childhood II. *Pediatr* 1973; 82:558-77.

Hyperthyroidism
1. Foley TP: Goiter in children. *Pediatr in Rev* 1984; 5:259-72.
2. Behrman R, Vaughan V: *Nelson Textbook of Pediatrics.* 13th ed., Chapter 19: The Endocrine System - Disorders of the Thyroid Gland. Philadelphia: W.B. Saunders Co., 1987; pp. 1199-1204.

Hypothryoidism
1. Fisher D: Hypothyroidism in childhood. *Pediatr in Rev* 1980; 2:67-74.
2. Foley TP: Goiter in children. *Pediatr in Rev* 1984; 5:259-72.
3. Behrman R, Vaughan V: *Nelson Textbook of Pediatrics*. 13th ed. Chapter 19: The Endocrine System - Disorders of the Thyroid Gland. Philadelphia: W.B. Saunders Co., 1987; pp. 1195-9.

Short Stature
1. Frasier S: Short stature in children. *Pediatr in Rev* 1981; 3:171-8.
2. Frawley T: Pituitary and adrenal disease. In Shen JTY: *The Clinical Practice of Adolescent Medicine*. NY: Appleton-Century Crofts, 1980; pp. 273-4.
3. Hofmann A: *Adolescent Medicine*. Reading, Mass: Addison-Wesley Publishing Co., 1983; pp. 170-2.
4. Root A, et al: Short stature-When is growth hormone indicated? *Contemp Pediatr* 1987; 4:26-56.

Gynecomastia
1. Neinstein LS: Adolescent Health Care: Chapter 10: *Gynecomastia*. Baltimore: Urban and Schwantzenberg, Inc., 1984; pp. 145-7.

Precocious Puberty, Premature Thelarche,and Premature Adrenarche
1. Emans SJ, Goldstein DP: *Pediatric and Adolescent Gynecology*. Boston: Little, Brown & Co., 1977; pp. 59-69.
2. Hofman A: *Adolescent Medicine*. Reading, Mass: Addison-Wesley Publishing Co., 1983; pp. 160-80.
3. Shen JTY: *The Clinical Practice of Adolescent Medicine*. NY: Appleton-Century Crofts, 1980; pp. 267-83.
4. Rosenfield RL: Androgen disorders in children: Too much, too early, too little, or too late. *Pediatr in Rev.* 1983; 5:147-156.
5. Cacciari E, et al: How many cases of true precocious puberty in girls are idiopathic? *J Pediatr* 1983; 357-60.
6. Mills JL, et al: Premature thelarche - Natural history and etiologic investigation. *AJDC* 1981; 135:743-5.

FEVER AND HEAT STRESS

A. Definition of Fever

Rectal temp >38° C (100.4° F). Rectal temp more reliable than oral temp. Rectal temp is approximately 0.6° C higher than oral temp and 1.1°C higher than axillary temp.

B. Fever is an important physiological sign of illness and is valuable in following the course of a disease as well as response to therapy.

Consequences of fever:
1. ↑HR, ↑ cardiac output
2. Anti-infection properties or effects
3. Malaise, discomfort, irritability (The disease or the fever?)

C. Not All Fevers Need Treatment

1. Why is symptomatic therapy possibly indicated?
   a. May reduce risk of febrile seizure.
   b. May decrease discomfort.
   c. May decrease energy expenditure in cardiovascular-compromised pt (e.g., pt with CHD or sickle cell disease).
2. Determine when symptomatic therapy is necessary and advise parents accordingly.

3. Educate parents that temperature won't "keep going up" if no treatment is given (T >41°C is rare), and that fever itself (<41°C) does not cause damage.
4. Treat the patient, not the number.

D. Treatment

1. Remove excess clothing and blankets. Hydrate with cool oral liquids.
2. Sponge with tepid water. Cold water is uncomfortable, and alcohol has potential risk of toxicity from inhalation.
3. Antipyretics
   a. Acetaminophen: Comparable to ASA as an antipyretic and less toxic in animals. Possible additive effect with sponging.
      1) Be certain parents understand difference in concentration of acetaminophen in drops vs. elixir (1 tsp elixir = 160 mg; 1 tsp drops = 500 mg).
         a) Tylenol drops = 100 mg/cc
         b) Elixir = 160 mg/5 cc
         c) Chewable tablets = 80 mg each
         d) Regular adult tablets/capsules = 325 mg each
         e) Extra strength = 500 mg each
         f) Suppository = 120, 300, 600 mg each
      2) Acetaminophen dose:
         a) 10-15 mg/kg/dose q 4-6 h or
         b) 60-80 mg/kg/ 24 hr per yr of age up to 5 yr
   b. Aspirin (ASA)-rarely indicated due to risk of Reye's syndrome
      1) Concentration of preparations
         a) Baby ASA = 75 mg
         b) Adult ASA = 300 mg; extra strength = 500 mg
         c) Suppository = 60, 300, 600 mg
      2) Dose: 10 mg/kg/dose q 4-6 h or
         1 baby ASA/yr up to age 5 yr

E. Evaluation of Febrile Patients

1. Infants under 8 weeks
   a. Almost <u>all</u> infants with temp > 38°C/100.4°F warrant full sepsis workup.
   b. Source will be identified in about 50% of cases (otitis meningitis, pneumonia, gastroenteritis). No source (?viral) in 50%.
   c. Usual procedure is sepsis w/u, admit, and start IV antibiotics pending culture results; however, this is <u>not</u> mandatory.
2. Older infants and children
   a. Most will turn out to have viral illnesses, but need to R/O treatable conditions such as strep, otitis, pneumonia, osteomyelitis, meningitis, UTI, bacteremia, etc.
   b. Urinalysis/urine culture indicated if no obvious source of fever. A negative urinalysis does not R/O UTI.
   c. PE unreliable to R/O pneumonia; need CXR.
   d. LP indicated with:
      1) Young infants
      2) Temperature. > 41°C
      3) Toxic appearance
      4) Abnormal neurologic exam
   e. Be alert to occult bacteremia (90% due to <u>Streptococcus pneumoniae</u>). Risk factors for bacteremia include:
      1) Age - 6-24 months
      2) Fever > 39°C
      3) WBC >15,000
      4) ESR > 30 mm/hr
      5) <u>Toxic appearance</u> - most important
   f. If patient is in high risk group for bacteremia, expectant Rx with ceftriaxone or ampicillin may be indicated (LP should be done prior to Rx), although supportive evidence is controversial.
   g. These patients need <u>close</u> F/U.

F. Heat Stress

1. The clinical features of heat-related illness are compared in the table.

	Heat Exhaustion	Heat Stroke
Onset	Often gradual	Usually acute
Temp	Normal or mild elevation	40.6°C or above
BP	Normal or slightly hypotensive	Hypotensive
Skin	Moist, clammy profuse sweating	Usually hot and dry but may be moist
CNS	Dizziness, headache, irritability, disorientation	Agitation, confusion seizures, lethargy, coma
GI	Nausea, vomiting	Vomiting, diarrhea
Serum Na	Normal or elevated	Elevated

2. Complications of heat stroke are outlined below:
   a. Cardiovascular: ECG changes, hypotension, myocardial dysfunction.
   b. Hematologic: DIC, fibrinolysis, thrombocytopenia.
   c. Hepatic: cholestasis,↑ liver enzymes, jaundice (often delayed 1-3 days).
   d. Metabolic: hypernatremia, hypoglycemia, hypokalemia, lactic acidosis.
   e. Renal: acute renal failure
3. Treatment
   a. Heat Exhaustion (heat collapse)
      1) Remove to cool environment - cover body with ice water - cooled towels.
      2) Replace fluid losses - orally if sensorium clear, otherwise, with IV fluids.
   b. Heat Stroke
      1) Treat as true emergency - transport patient to nearest emergency medical facility.

2) During transport, remove all clothing and cool with cold water towels.
3) In ER, place patient in ice water bath and rapidly cool to a core temp of 38.3°C-38.8°C.
4) Massage extremities to increase peripheral blood flow.
5) Replace fluid and electrolyte losses with Ringer's lactate.
6) Supplemental O_2.
7) Monitor rectal temp and ECG.
8) Monitor and treat complications.

DO NOT USE ANTIPYRETICS OR DRUGS TO PREVENT SHIVERING.

N.B. The diagnosis of heat stroke should be considered, regardless of climate, when acute encephalopathy in infants is associated with high fever.

References

Fever

1. Carroll WL, et al: Treatment of occult bacteremia: A prospective randomized clinical trial. *Pediatr* 1983; 72:608.
2. Caspe W, Chamudes O, Louie B: The evaluation and treatment of the febrile infant. *Ped Inf Dis* 1983; 2:131.
3. Cone TE Jr: Diagnosis and treatment: Children with fevers. *Pediatr* 43: 1969; 290.
4. Crain EF, Shelov SP: Febrile infants: Predictors of bacteremia. *J Pediatr* 1982; 101:686.
5. Klein J, Schlesinger P, Karasic R: Management of the febrile infant three months of age or younger. *Ped Inf Dis* 1984; 3:75.
6. Kluger M: Fever. *Pediatr* 66: 1980; 720.
7. McCarthy P: What tests are indicated for the child under 2 with fever? *Pediatrics in Review,* 1979; 1:52.
8. Roberts KB, Charney E, Sweren RT, et al: Urinary tract infections with unexplained fever. *J Pediatr* 1983; 103:864.
9. Schmitt BD: Fever phobia. Misconceptions of parents about fevers. *AJDC* 1972; 123: 204.
10. Stern RC: Pathophysiologic basis for symptomatic treatment of fever. *Pediatr* 59: 1977; 59: 92.
11. Steele RW, et al. Oral antipyretic therapy. Evaluation of aspirin-acetaminophen combination. *Am J Dis Child* 1972; 123S:204.

Heat Stress

1. Bacon C, Scott D, Jones P: Heat stroke in well-wrapped infants. *Lancet* 1979; 1:422.
2. Danks DM, Webb DW, Allen J: Heat illness in infants and young children. *Brit Med J* 1962; 2:287.
3. Rosenstein BJ: The twin perils of heat exhausation and heatstroke. *Contemp Pediatr* May 1986; 46-52.

7

GASTROINTESTINAL DISORDERS

A. Abdominal Pain

1. Abdominal pain may be acute or chronic/recurrent (at least 3 episodes in 3 mo). It may represent surgical, medical, and emotional conditions.
   Chronic/recurrent abdominal pain will occur in approximately 10% of children 5-10 yr old; however, less than 10% of these will have an organic basis (frequently genitourinary) for the pain.
2. The history should be tailored to the circumstances of the pain (acute vs. chronic/recurrent).
   a. Where is the pain located; does it radiate? Is it cramping, sharp, dull, constant, or intermittent?
   b. Does the pain make the child cry or abandon his usual activity? Does it occur at particular times of the day or certain days of the week? Does it awaken him from sleep? What is its relation to meals?
   c. How long does the pain last?
   d. What are precipitating events, factors, or medications (including prescriptions, over-the-counter preparations, home remedies) that relieve the pain?
   e. What is the child's diet?
   f. Does he have any allergies or food intolerances? Which ones?

g. Is he on any medications? Which ones?

h. Does he have a chronic medical condition? Which one?

i. Has he ever had a diagnosed GI medical problem or GI surgery (elaborate)?

j. Is the pain accompanied by anorexia, nausea, vomiting, bloating, flatulence, diarrhea, or constipation?

k. Are non-GI symptoms present (fever, sore throat, rash, cough, headache, joint symptoms, etc)?

l. Is there a history of trauma (elaborate)?

m. Do other family members have similar symptoms?

n. In the adolescent female, is there a history of vaginal discharge or bleeding?

o. Has there been a change in the child's environment (home, friends, school) or behavior (poor school performance, apathy, argumentativeness, etc.)?

3. A complete PE is essential with special emphasis on the abdomen.

a. With the patient supine, the abdomen should be inspected for evidence of trauma (bruises, lacerations, etc,) chronic medical conditions (café au lait spots/neurofibromatosis; ash-leaf spots/ tuberous sclerosis), rashes or petechiae, asymmetries, or distension. Is there a scaphoid abdomen or is a hernia present? Is there reverse peristalsis?

b. Palpation of the abdomen should be done to elicit evidence of tenderness (including rebound), masses, or organomegaly. Are fluid waves present?

c. Detection of tenderness may be difficult in a crying, frightened child; sometimes, examination with the child sitting on his parent's lap may lessen his fear. In addition, if a child reports that "everything hurts" but doesn't act appropriately, palpation with the stethoscope ("I'm going to listen to you now") might help to sort out real areas (if any) of tenderness. The child in real pain will say "ow," flinch, jump, blink his eyes, tear, etc., if stethoscope palpation is painful.

d. Percussion of the abdomen is performed to determine the liver span, areas of dullness (shifting?), and overall tympanicity.

e. Auscultation should be used to determine the presence and quality (hypo-normo-hyperactive, tinkles, rushes) of bowel sounds in each quadrant.

f. One should try to elicit the presence of peritoneal signs (obturator/psoas).

g. Unless the diagnosis is felt to be an uncomplicated gastroenteritis, a rectal exam should be performed to detect masses, tenderness, hard stool, etc.

h. If the patient is an adolescent girl, a pelvic exam should be considered.

i. Finally, any patient with abdominal pain should be observed (1) walking, (2) climbing onto the exam table, (3) getting down from the table, and (4) interacting with both parents and staff to gain some insight into the degree of incapacitation or emotional overlay that may be present.

4. Selected causes of abdominal pain

a. Infectious: Viral gastroenteritis, bacterial enteritis, food poisoning (especially <u>Staphylococcus aureus, Salmonella), Clostridium difficile</u> infection, parasite infestation, hepatitis, pneumonia (basilar), urinary tract infection, pelvic inflammatory disease, Group A streptococcal infection.

b. Surgical: Obstruction, stenosis, malrotation, intussusception, Meckel's diverticulum, appendicitis, cholelithiasis, tumors.

c. Medical: Cholecystitis, pancreatitis, renal calculi, ulcerative colitis, regional enteritis, Hirschsprung's disease, constipation, gastroesophageal reflux, ulcer (gastric and duodenal), ab-

dominal migraine, indigestion, allergic reactions to foods, medication use (especially erythromycin), porphyria, lactase deficiency, sickle cell crisis, pancreatitis.
  d. Trauma: Blows to the abdomen or back, falls.
  e. Emotional: Depression, anxiety, school phobia, irritable bowel (spastic colon).
5. Laboratory tests are dictated by the history and physical findings.
  a. If an acute surgical condition is suspected, a cbc with diff, ESR, serum chemistries (electrolytes, BUN, creatinine, glucose), and a type and crossmatch are indicated in conjunction with radiographic studies of the abdomen, a stool guaiac, and a U/A.
  b. The same studies may be indicated with blunt abdominal trauma; an ultrasound or CT study may be needed to locate the site and extent of hematomas, etc.
  c. If pancreatitis is suspected, a serum amylase should be obtained.
  d. If stones are suspected, a U/A and radiologic (or ultrasound) studies of the abdomen may be diagnostic.
  e. When inflammatory bowel disease is being considered, a cbc with diff, ESR, stool guaiac, and culture, and flat and upright abdominal films may be helpful initially; sigmoidoscopy and biopsy will confirm the diagnosis.
  f. When gastroesophageal reflux is suspected, a stool guaiac is obtained; diagnosis is confirmed by pH measurement of the lower esophagus, measurement of lower esophageal sphincter pressure, or endoscopy. A barium swallow may be normal if reflux is only intermittent. A barium swallow often shows reflux in young infants and should not be the only basis for a diagnosis of pathologic GER.

g. Lactase deficiency is diagnosed by an abnormal breath hydrogen test.

h. When uncomplicated viral gastroenteritis is suspected, no laboratory tests (except, perhaps, a U/A) are mandatory. However, when a bacterial enteritis is suspected, a stool guaiac, methylene blue exam of the stool (to detect white blood cells), and stool culture are indicated; a cbc with diff and blood cultures should be obtained if the child is ill.

i. If parasitic infestation is suspected, a fresh stool sample for ova and parasites should be obtained.

j. The possibility of hepatitis necessitates a U/A, stool examination, serum bilirubin, liver function tests, and hepatitis serology screen.

k. Group A strep pharyngitis, urinary tract infection, and pelvic inflammatory disease require appropriate cultures.

l. The child with suspected emotion-related pain should have a paucity of studies: a U/A (to R/O occult urinary tract infection), a stool guaiac, culture and sample for ova/parasites (to R/O occult infection), and <u>perhaps</u> a cbc with diff and ESR.

6. Treatment is directed at the underlying cause of the pain.

a. Surgical problems are treated accordingly.

b. Proven infections are treated with the appropriate antibiotic or antimicrobial.

c. Inflammatory bowel disease responds to proper diet (including iron supplementation), symptomatic relief of diarrhea, sulfasalazine (intially 250-500 mg qid to a maxium of 2-8 g/d), steroids (prednisone 1-2 mg/kg to a maximum of 60 mg/d).

d. Individuals with lactase deficiency will benefit from a lactose-free diet or exogenous lactase replacement (available in tablets).

e. Patients with reflux benefit from small, frequent meals (rather than infrequent, large ones), sitting upright or sleeping at a 45° angle after eating, avoidance of late evening meals, metaclopramide or bethanecol and cimetidine.

f. Patients with ulcers benefit from elimination of foods which seem to exacerbate symptoms, ingestion of antacids, H_2 blockers, and relaxation techniques.

g. Children with emotion-related abdominal pain (and their parents) require patience, and reassurance. Psychotherapy may be indicated in children with handicapping pain whether organic or not.

B. Anal Fissure

1. An anal fissure is a break in the anal skin or in the rectal mucosa.

   a. Such breaks are caused by passing (with straining) hard stools or by the insertion of objects (suppositories, thermometers, wedges of soap) in the anus in an attempt to stimulate stool passage.

   b. Blood is either on the outside of a hard stool or is mixed in a linear pattern in a looser stool.

   c. Fissures are particularly common in infants.

   d. The child is otherwise well although he may cry during stooling.

   e. A history of constipation or attempts to stimulate stooling may be obtained.

2. With the child supine, the buttocks are spread to stretch the anus. The fissure's location is compared to the position of the hands on a clock ("fissure at 8 o'clock"). A proctoscopic exam is performed to ascertain the presence of internal fissures.

3. Treatment is simple: Soften the stools (see Section D,"Constipation"), cease the insertion of objects into the anus, keep the area as clean as possible, and apply petroleum jelly locally with each diaper change.

C. Gastrointestinal Bleeding

1. Gastrointestinal bleeding can occur anywhere in the GI tract. Such bleeding may be acute or chronic, gross or microscopic, manifested in vomitus (hematemesis), in stool (melena: gross blood), or in both.

2. Important historical information includes:
   a. The onset and duration of the bleeding,
   b. Color (bright vs dark red),
   c. Rate (brisk vs gradual),
   d. Possible antecedent events (e.g., epistaxis),
   e. Presence of clots,
   f. Description of the vomiting or diarrhea (whichever is appropriate),
   g. The child's condition or mental status (normal vs semiconscious/shocky),
   h. The presence of pain, location, radiation),
   i. The presence of previous GI trauma (e.g., lye ingestions), surgery, or medical condition,
   j. The presence of a chronic medical condition (e.g., hemosiderosis) or medication use (which?),
   k. Hematological problem,
   l. The possibility of an ingestion (elaborate as to what, how much, and when).
   m. Remember, many episodes of "red" vomitus or diarrhea are not secondary to bleeding but instead are the result of ingestion of red fluids or foods; thus, a dietary history of the previous 24-48 hours is necessary for all patients.

3. The PE should be complete. Particular attention should be paid to:
   a. The vital signs (evidence of shock, orthostatic changes, infections),
   b. The child's mental status (in pain, in shock), spontaneous movements (evidence of peritonitis, surgical abdomen),
   c. Skin (petechiae, purpura, trauma),
   d. Mouth and nose (evidence of previous bleeding),
   e. Abdomen (distension, areas of tenderness, organomegaly, presence of masses, quality and loca-

tion of bowel sounds),
    f. Rectal exam (fissures, hemorrhoids, trauma).
    g. Is active bleeding occuring now? From what orifice?
4. Unless the source of the bleeding is clearly oral bleeding, epistaxis, anal fissure, or hemorrhoids, a cbc with diff, platelet count, and coagulation studies should be obtained.
    a. Urine should be examined for the presence of blood.
    b. If the diarrhea is bloody, a methylene blue stain of the stool and a stool culture should be performed.
    c. A sepsis workup may need to be considered for certain patients, especially neonates.
    d. Similarly, a CXR may be indicated if the respiratory exam is abnormal.
    e. If the child is actively bleeding, in shock, or has an acute surgical abdomen, other laboratory tests may be necessary (clotting studies, serum electrolytes, BUN, creatinine, type and crossmatch, etc).
5. Some causes of GI bleeding
    a. Swallowed blood (newborn S/P delivery, infant nursing at cracked/bleeding breast, epistaxis, oral/pharyngeal trauma or bleeding): amount of bleeding may be variable.
    b. Esophagitis/gastritis due to ingestion of a corrosive or iron/aspirin overdose: amount of bleeding may be variable.
    c. Esophageal varices due to portal hypertension: massive or chronic, low-grade bleeding.
    d. Esophageal tear due to trauma or foreign body ingestion: variable bleeding (usually large).
    e. Esophageal inflammation due to hiatal hernia or chalasia: variable bleeding.
    f. Gastritis due to intractable vomiting (viral infection, S/P ipecac use, anorexia nervosa, pyloric stenosis: small amount of bleeding.

g. Hemorrhagic gastritis of the newborn due to sepsis, CNS disease, overwhelming systemic illness: massive bleeding.

h. Gastric ulcer/duodenal ulcer (midepigastric pain, vomiting): variable bleeding (may be massive).

i. Stress ulcer due to sepsis, CNS disease: large amount of bleeding.

j. Gastric outlet obstruction (especially pyloric stenosis): small amount of bleeding.

k. Enteritis due to infection (certain viruses, especially rotavirus; <u>Salmonella, Shigella,</u> invasive <u>E. coli, Campylobacter, Clostridium difficile</u> overgrowth S/P antibiotic therapy): variable bleeding.

l. Intestinal surgical disorders (volvulus, obstruction, intussusception (currant jelly stools), Meckel's diverticulum, polyps, masses, perforation due to foreign body ingestion): variable bleeding, usually large.

m. Intestinal hemangiomas: variable bleeding.

n. Infantile milk allergy: variable bleeding.

o. Hemosiderosis: may be massive bleeding.

p. Ingestions, especially iron or aspirin: may be massive bleeding.

q. Henoch-Schonlein purpura (hemorrhagic rash, melena, abdominal pain, arthritis, hematuria): variable bleeding, may be marked.

r. Hemolytic-uremic syndrome (bloody diarrhea, renal failure, anemia, thrombocytopenia, CNS disturbances): may be massive bleeding.

s. Ulcerative colitis (bloody diarrhea, weight loss, abdominal pain, arthritis, uveitis): variable bleeding.

t. Regional enteritis (bloody diarrhea, weight loss, abdominal pain, growth failure, anemia, arthritis, fever): variable bleeding, may be marked.

u. Anal Fissure: small amount of bleeding.

v. Hemorrhoids: small to moderate bleeding.

w. Proctitis due to gonorrhea: usually small amount of bleeding.

x. Hematologic disorders (Vitamin K deficiency in the neonate, aplastic anemia, leukemia, thrombocytopenia, hemophilia): may be massive bleeding.

y. Sepsis, especially due to N. meningitidis.

6. The child with moderate to massive upper GI bleeding should remain NPO.

a. A nasogastric tube is inserted and gastric lavage is instituted using normal saline; lavage until the return is clear. Leave the tube in place (intermittent suction). If active bleeding continues, the child may need to go to the operating room. Diagnostic endoscopy is usually indicated.

b. Surgical conditions should be corrected.

c. Known infections should be treated with the appropriate antibiotic.

d. Iron ingestion is treated with fluids and electrolytes (and base, if pH <7.1) and with IV deferoxamine if the serum iron is >500 (see pg. 153).

e. ASA ingestion is treated with fluids, electrolytes, and base, if pH <7.1; dialysis may be necessary (see pg. 155).

f. Uncomplicated Henoch-Schonlein purpura can be treated with NSAIDs.

g. Patients with milk allergy and hemoderosis require elimination of milk from their diets.

h. The managements of ulcerative colitis, regional enteritis, anal fissure, hemolytic-uremic syndrome, and foreign body ingestion are discussed elsewhere.

i. Hemorrhoids are treated by keeping the stools soft and applying epinephricaine to them; recalcitrant cases may require proctoscopic evaluation.

D. Constipation

1. Constipation is the condition in which the child

fails to completely empty the colon with bowel movements. Stools are often hard, difficult to pass, and infrequent.

a. The usual cause of constipation is dietary indiscretion (diet high in dairy products and complex carbohydrates or low in fiber/bulk; insufficient fluid intake).

b. Starvation or intractable vomiting may lead to infrequent stooling.

c. Resistance to toilet training and psychological problems may lead to constipation in the absence of organic pathology.

d. Irritation of the anus (rashes, fissures) may cause stooling avoidance.

e. Miscellaneous causes of constipation include Hirschsprung's disease, hypothyroidism, and certain medications, especially antidepressants.

2. Important historical information includes:

a. The onset, duration, and recurrences of the constipation; most patients with Hirschsprung's disease will have a history of abnormal stools starting in the first month of life.

b. The individual's usual stool pattern and daily diet,

c. The age of successful toilet-training (if applicable),

d. The presence of anorexia or vomiting,

e. The presence of diarrhea or fecal spotting alternating with periods of constipation (Hirschsprung's disease, encopresis),

f. The presence of anal lesions, fissures, rashes,

g. Psychological difficulties,

h. Medication use (which ones?),

i. Hypothyroidism (see pp. 56-58)

3. The PE is usually normal except for the presence of hard stool palpable in the lower abdomen or in the rectum. The anus and surrounding area should be examined for rashes, lesions, and fissures.

4. Most children with constipation require no laboratory tests. If hypothyroidism is suspected, a T_3/T_4

and TSH are indicated. A rectal mucosal biopsy will confirm the diagnosis of Hirschsprung's disease.

5. Treatment

   a. The constipated child with impaction should receive an enema (Fleets or Pediatric Fleets depending on the child's age) and a stool softener (Colace) or a peristalsis-inducer (Senokot) orally.

   b. The constipated child without impaction does not require such measures.

   c. The diet should be improved; specifically, this involves (1) increasing fluid intake, (2) decreasing the amount of complex carbohydrates (especially junk food), (3) increasing the amount of fiber and bulk (leafy vegetables work well), and (4) daily ingestion of apple juice or pineapple juice (undiluted).

   d. Senokot, Colace or lactulose should be reserved for children (not infants) in whom dietary measures are insufficient.

   e. The routine use of laxatives and enemas is discouraged.

   f. Anal fissures which can be associated with constipation are discussed on pg. 80.

   g. Battles over toilet-training and emotional dysfunctioning require patience and counseling; the latter may also require psychotherapy.

   h. Hirshchsprung's disease should be managed in consultation with a pediatric surgeon or gastroenterologist; affected children require emotional support and, occasionally, psychotherapy.

E. Diarrhea (i.e., Increased Frequency and Water Content of Stools)

1. The history should elicit the duration (chronic, acute, recurrent), frequency, amount, and consistency. Compare to patient's usual stooling pattern.

   a. What are the characteristics of the stool (bloody,

       mucous, black, pale, greasy, foul-smelling, etc.)?
  b. Determine the diet history (lactose intolerance, celiac disease, food poisoning), medication history (has pt been on antibiotics?), and travel history.
  c. Is there fever, vomiting, anorexia, cramps, headache, rash, lethargy, or a decrease in urination?
  d. Can patient tolerate oral liquids?
  e. Has there been a recent exposure to others with diarrhea or with a H/O salmonella or to food handlers in family/friends?
  f. Is the child in day care? Are day-care contacts ill?
2. The PE should assess the child's vital signs, weight, appearance (toxic vs. well), degree of hydration, and perfusion.
  a. Other foci of infection (ear, throat, lungs, urine) should be checked.
  b. Emphasize the abdominal exam, the skin (turgor, mucous membranes, purpura, other exanthem), and the neurologic exam (alertness, activity, tone, seizures).
  c. A rectal exam may be necessary if the diarrheal illness is more than mild.
3. Laboratory assessment of diarrhea includes
  a. Stool exam: Evaluate for blood, mucus, appearance, and consistency;use methylene blue stain of stool smear to look for PMN's. Culture for bacterial etiology if you suspect salmonella, shigella, or if the child is toxic appearing or has a high fever. Examine for parasites if indicated; and stool for <u>Clostridium</u> toxin if indicated.
  b. Urine: Dipstick sp. gr.; microscropic. Culture if indicated.
  c. Blood: Obtain cbc, electrolytes, BUN, culture when indicated.
4. Etiology
  a. Acute diarrhea
    1)Viral:
      a) Rotavirus

- Frequent cause of acute diarrhea in infants often preceded or accompanied by vomiting
- Occurs year-round but usually in winter
- Incubation 1-3 d; duration 5-8 d
- May have fever and vomiting
- may have ↓ HCO_3
- Dx: ELISA.

b) Enterovirus
  - Occurs usually in summer
  - Dx: ELISA

c) Adenovirus:
  - Year-round occurrence
  - Causes GI/respiratory illness symptoms
  - Dx: ELISA

d) Norwalk:
  - Epidemic
  - Self-limited (24-48 hr)
  - Dx: Electron microscopy of stool (research purposes only)

2) Bacterial (accounts for 20% of acute GE):

a) <u>Shigella</u>
  - Seasonal peak-July to September
  - Peak incidence 1-5 yr
  - Invades gut wall; bloody, mucoid stools
  - May be associated with febrile seizures (↑ temp)
  - Vomiting not prominent
  - Polys in stool
  - ↑ Bands in blood
  - Treatment: ampicillin (NOT amoxicillin), 75 mg/kg/d divided qid or Trimethoprim-sulfamethoxazole, 1 cc/kg/d (or 8mg/kg/d TMP, 40 mg/kg/d SMZ) divided bid

b) Salmonella:
  - Any age, but higher under 1 yr
  - Invades gut wall; bloody, mucoid stools
  - ± temp elevation
  - Vomiting not prominent
  - Polys in stool

- Incubation 6-48 hr; 2-5 d course
- Organism may be shed in stool for months
- Transient bacteremia in 20-40% of infants with <u>Salmonella</u> GE.
- For uncomplicated GE, no treatment is necessary
- Antibiotic indicated for infants <3 months (increased incidence of complications) and for highly febrile patients (enteric fever picture)

c) E. coli:
- Either invades mucosa (bloody stool) or produces an enterotoxin

d) Campylobacter fetus:
- Invasive (blood and mucus); in neonates may cause bloody diarrhea without other clinical manifestations
- Severe abdominal cramps
- Vomiting/dehydration uncommon
- ↑ Incidence in summer
- Usually resolves spontaneously, but if need to treat, use erythromycin, 50 mg/kg/d divided qid

e) Yersinia enterocolitica:
- Mucoid stools
- Polys frequently present in stools
- Severe abdominal pain possible
- Diarrhea x 1-2 wk
- Often mimics appendicitis
- Treament: not usually indicated for infections confined to GI tract

3) Noninfectious:
a) Acute poisoning (Fe, Hg, Pb, fluoride)
b) Antibiotic induced (Ampicillin in particular); pseudomembranous enterocolitis caused by <u>Clostridium difficile</u> overgrowth after antibiotic use
c) Hemolytic-Uremic syndrome (hemolysis; thrombocytopenia; melena; hematuria;

renal failure; CNS symptoms such as seizures, behavior changes, coma, and shock)
   d) Toxic shock syndrome (mediated by <u>S. aureus</u> toxin; associated with tampon use); osteomyelitis; abscess; pneumonia, GU infection; S/sx include fever, diarrhea, hyperemic mucous membranes, macular red rash that is generalized, hypotension, and shock)
   e) Intussusception (paroxysms of pain, bloody diarrhea - currant jelly stools, irritability OR pale, apathetic state)
b. Chronic diarrhea:
   1) Infectious causes:
      a) Amebiasis
         • Chronic diarrhea, lower abdominal pain, or perianal abscess
         • May be asymptomatic
         • ± stool polys
         • ± fever (recurrent)
         • Mucoid stool
         • Treatment: (Iodoquinol 40 mg/kg/d divided tid x 20d (max = 2 g/d) or paromomycin 25-35 mg/kg/d divided tid x 5-10d
      b) Giardiasis
         • Chronic diarrhea or lower abdominal pain
         • May be asymptomatic or have frequent relapses
         • Treatment: quinacrine HCl (Atabrine)
         > 8 yr - 1 tab(0.1g)   tid x 5d
         4-8yr - 1/2 tab   tid x 5d
         < 4 yr - 1/2 tab   bid x 5d
                  OR
         metronidazole x 10d children 5 mg/kg/d
                                 adults 10 mg/kg/d
      c) Occasionally, <u>E. coli, Salmonella,</u> and <u>Yersinia</u> diarrhea may become persistent or recurrent.

2) Non-infectious causes
   a) Ulcerative colitis (fever, abdominal pain, diarrhea - may be bloody, arthralgias, arthritis, growth failure)
   b) Regional enteritis (fever, abdominal pain, arthritis, diarrhea - may be bloody, growth failure)
   c) Hirschsprung's disease (constipation alternating with diarrhea or fecal spotting)
   d) Lactase deficiency
   e) Metabolic/malabsorption diseases (such as cystic fibrosis, disaccharidase deficiencies, celiac disease, etc.)
   f) Irritable colon
   g) Encopresis
   h) Food allergies

5. Treatment

   There is controversy regarding the most appropriate way to manage outpatient acute diarrhea. The following are guidelines. The goal is to correct hydration and electrolyte imbalance and maximize nutrition.

   a. D/C lactose-containing formulas and milk:

   Older children may be able to tolerate solid diet plus oral glucose-electrolyte solution. Breast-fed infants appear to tolerate continuation of nursing. Children who continue some solids and breast-fed infants who continue nursing may have slight increase in stooling initially, but no prolongation of total duration of diarrhea. If an infant is not dehydrated or is only mildly so and is tolerating oral feeds, he may be managed with full-strength soy formula or oral electrolyte solutions (see below).

   b. Oral glucose-electrolyte solutions (OGES)

   1) If an infant can take po fluids and is mildly to moderately dehydrated (<8%), rehydration may proceed with OGES.

   Rehydration with OGES can be carried out

even in patients with mild to moderate hypo- or hypernatremia.

Some OGES are low in Na concentration (30 mEq/L). In mild, self-limited diarrhea, this lower Na concentration is usually not a problem. Continue OGES x 12-36 hr.

2) If child is moderately to severely dehydrated (>7-8%) may need admission for appropriate replacement of fluids and electrolytes. This may be done orally, if tolerated, or intravenously.

c. Dehydration:

1) If child is severely dehydrated (>10%): Rapid volume expansion by IV of Ringer's lactate (20 cc/kg/h) x 1-2 hr. Calculate estimated deficits of water and electrolytes. Replace deficits over 4-8 hr. Give pt his/her maintenance and cover ongoing losses for that same time period.

2) After this initial period, continue calculated maintenance and ongoing loss therapy. Pt may be given oral glucose-electrolyte solution after initial 4-8 hr therapy if able to tolerate. Continue x 12-36 hr.

Composition of Solutions Available for Oral Therapy			
	Lytren	Pedialyte	WHO Std.
Na (meq/L)	50	45	90
K (meq/L)	25	20	20
Cl (meq/L)	45	35	80
HCO3 or citrate (meq/L)	30	30	30
Glucose (grams/L)	20	25	20

3) Never treat diarrhea with 1/2 strength Pedialyte or Lytren; those dilutions don't even supply <u>maintenance</u> electrolytes for someone <u>without</u> diarrhea.

4) Other frequently used "clear liquids" (e.g., apple juice, cola, ginger ale, Kool-Aid) are inadequate in electrolyte composition for rehydration or maintenance therapy, and should not be utilized in mainstay of therapy except for very brief intervals or as "free water" replacement.

5) Homemade solutions are fraught with all the hazards of errors in measuring and mixing, and their use should be discouraged.

d. Advance diet to non-lactose formula for infants who are not breast feeding (e.g., Isomil) and to BRATS diet (<u>B</u>ananas, <u>R</u>ice, <u>A</u>pplesauce, <u>T</u>oast, <u>S</u>altines) x 24 hr. Continue to normalize diet as tolerated.

e. Treatment for underlying cause of diarrhea:

1) Treatment for bacterial and parasitic infections includes the use of the appropriate antimicrobial.

2) Pseudomembranous colitis due to <u>Clostridium difficile</u> is treated by discontinuation of the offending antimicrobial, restoration of fluid and electrolyte balance, and vancomycin 40-60 mg/kg/d x 7-10 d.

3) Other antibiotic associated diarrheas are treated by discontinuing the drug.

4) Hemolytic uremic syndrome is treated with appropriate fluid and electrolytes by intravenous infusion, blood transfusions (if necessary), seizure control, and management of increased intracranial pressure.

5) Toxic shock syndrome should be treated with nafcillin or oxacillin 100-200 mg/kg/d, IV fluids, vasopressors to maintain a normal blood pressure, and ventilatory support, if necessary.

6) Intussusception is treated by hydrastatic reduction with barium enema or surgery (unsuccessful hydrastatic reduction, symptoms > 2 d, recurrent episodes, obstruction, or peritonitis).

F. Encopresis

1. Encopresis is recurrent fecal incontinence in the absence of organic disease. About 1% of 7-8 yr olds (the peak age) are affected, with a male-female ratio of 3:1. Approximately half of the children have never been completely bowel trained. A single episode of fecal incontinence should not be regarded as encopresis.

   a. Hypotheses on possible etiologies include premature or coercive toilet training, fear of defecation due to previous "accidents" or pain as would occur with an anal fissure, mental retardation, and isolated areas of neurodevelopmental delay.

   b. Organic lesions that can cause encopresis include those discussed under "Chronic Diarrhea" and several others, such as central or peripheral nervous system disease, defects in rectal or anal musculature, chronic constipation with resultant overflow, and chronic laxative or enema use.

2. Important historical information includes

   a. The onset and duration of the problem

   b. Current and previous stooling patterns

   c. Age of attainment of bowel control

   d. Appearance and consistency of stools

   e. The presence of constipation

   f. Chronic enema or laxative use

   g. Patterns of growth

   h. Psychosocial, emotional, familial, and scholastic assessments

3. The PE is usually normal. Emphasis should be placed on the neurologic exam and abdominal/

rectal exams. The anal tone should be normal (patulous if chronic enema use), and the rectal vault should be of normal size with feces present.

4. The possibility of organic disease should be obvious from the history and physical exam; if suspected, the workup is as discussed in "Chronic Diarrhea."

   a. A U/A and urine culture may demonstrate an occult urinary tract infection (2° to chronic constipation).

   b. Serum chemistries, ESR, cbc, and radiographic studies are usually normal in children with true encopresis.

5. Treatment of encopresis includes diet manipulation, colon evacuation with enemas or laxatives, establishment of (and reward for) a normal defecation pattern, reassurance, patience, counseling, and occasionally, psychotherapy.

G. Gastroesophageal Reflux

1. Gastroesophageal reflux (GER) is the return of stomach contents into the esophagus due to an incompetent lower esophageal sphincter. This incompetence may be due to immaturity (as in infants), esophageal disease, obstructive lung disease, or to overdistension of the stomach (due to overeating). A small degree of reflux after overeating is probably universal. GER may be accompanied by effortless vomiting (infants), aspiration pneumonia (infants), apnea (infants) belching, esophagitis (all ages), and mid-epigastric pain. Pain is worse after eating, especially if the patient is supine; in contrast, the pain of an ulcer, which is similarly located, is relieved by eating, especially in older children and adolescents.

2. In infants with suspected GER, the following questions are helpful.

   a. Is the infant vomiting (forceful projection) or "spitting up"?

    b. When does this occur (i.e., how long after a meal)?

    c. How is the infant fed (sitting up, lying down)? In what position is he placed after feeding? Does the position make a diffrence as to whether he is likely to spit-up?

    d. Is he a rapid eater?

    e. How much (and what kind of) formula does he take with each feeding? What other foods are ingested?

    f. Does he seem hungry?

    g. Is he gaining weight?

    h. What does the vomitus look like? Is it green- or red-tinged?

    i. Does the infant wheeze, cough, or turn blue? When? Has he ever had pneumonia? When?

    j. Are there feeding difficulties (elaborate)?

    k. Does he have fever or diarrhea? (Elaborate the time and height of fever and the onset, duration, and appearance of diarrhea.)

    l. Is he on any medications? Which one(s)? N.B. Theophylline may worsen GER.

    m. Have any over-the-counter preparations or home remedies been used to stop the vomiting? Which ones?

    n. In the older patient - where is the pain, if any, located and does it radiate? What is its relation to eating and lying down? What precipitates it; what causes relief?

    o. Is the child a rapid eater? Does he belch?

    p. Is the pain accompanied by fever, vomiting, diarrhea (if yes, elaborate further)?

    q. Has he ever vomited blood?

    r. Does pain interfere with his activities? Does it awaken him from sleep?

3. The PE is usually normal. Young infants, however, may present with failure-to-thrive, or, rarely, with torticollis (Sandifer's syndrome).

4. If significant vomiting, diarrhea, or failure-to-thrive is present, certain laboratory tests are useful

to secure a diagnosis.
  a. The individual with GER (but without failure-to-thrive) will usually have a normal cbc and serum chemistries, except for those individuals (especially infants) with significant reflux who may be alkalotic and hypochloremic.
  b. If the chest exam is abnormal, a CXR (to R/O aspiration pneumonia) is indicated.
  c. The diagnosis of mild reflux is made by the characteristic history. In moderate to severe reflux (especially if accompanied by failure-to-thrive or pulmonary symptoms), the diagnosis of GER may be confirmed by pH monitoring of the lower esophagus, measurement of lower esophageal sphincter pressure, or esophagoscopy (looking for evidence of esophagitis).
  d. A barium swallow may be normal since reflux may be only intermittent.
5. Treatment of the infant with GER includes small, frequent feedings in the upright position, thickened formula with cereal, and maintenance of a prone head-up position after feeding.
  a. If these measures fail, a trial of bethanecol (9 mg/m^2/24 h divided tid) or metaclopramide (0.1 mg/kg/dose prior to meals) may be efficacious in relieving the symptoms.
  b. If esophagitis is present, antacids might be useful.
  c. If medical management fails, fundoplication may be necessary.
  d. Treatment of the older child with GER includes small, frequent meals, maintenance of an upright position after meals, eating slowly, and no meals after 7 PM. An H$_2$ blocker (cimetidine or ranitidine) may be necessary.

H. Foreign Body (FB) Ingestion

1. The most common FBs ingested by children are metal objects (especially coins), buttons, small parts of toys, hair, tablets, and button batteries.

2. FB's that lodge in the esophagus may cause dysphagia, mid-sternal pain or fullness, gagging, choking, cough, or respiratory embarrassment.
   a. Diagnosis is by PA and lateral radiographs of the chest and neck.
   b. Location of the FB is usually in the upper esophagus (C4 level).
   c. Removal may be accomplished in two ways: (1) during esophagoscopy in the operating room, or (2) by using a #8-#14 Foley catheter in the emergency room. (A deflated catheter is passed into the sedated child's nose and into the esophagus; the balloon is inflated; the FB is removed by traction on the catheter.)
3. FB's that pass into the stomach will generally pass out of the body in 2-10 days. A radiograph should be obtained when the child first presents to localize the object's position. If the object does not pass in 10 days or if GI symptoms occur, the child should return for evaluation (and possibly treatment). Emetics and cathartics should not be used.

I. Parasites

1. Pinworms
   a. Diagnosis
      1) Intense pruritus ani especially at night; vulvo-vaginitis, UTI, irritability. No eosinophilia.
      2) Worms may be seen in rectal area or stool and lay eggs in anal skinfolds or vaginal introitus.
      3) Cellophane tape test: Press tape to perianal area (best in evening before going to bed). Mount tape over a drop of toluene on a glass slide and look for ova with a microscope.
   b. Treatment
      1) Often best to also treat other children at home. Some advise treating the entire family; make sure mother isn't pregnant.
      2) Launder bed clothes and undergarments. Make sure children sleep in underwear to avoid

contact of fingers with anus.
3) Medication
  a) Mebendazole (Vermox); same dose for all ages; 100 mg x 1. Not much experience in children <2 yr. Contraindicated in pregnant women.
  b) Pyrantel pamoate (Antiminth) 11 mg/kg to maximum of 1 gm; give in a single dose.
  c) Pyrvinium pamoate (Povan) 5 mg/kg in single dose to 250 mg. May cause GI upset, stain stools red.
  d) Piperazine citrate (Antepar) 50 mg/kg to maximum of 2 gm daily x 7 d.
c. Consider retreatment in 2 wk. Chance of reinfestation is very high.

J. **Vomiting**
  1. The history should differentiate between real vomiting and "spitting-up."
     a. Important questions about vomiting relate to its frequency, severity, appearance (blood or bile tinged), amount, time of occurrence, duration, projectile nature.
     b. What has the child taken by mouth (foods, medicines, poison)?
     c. How have the parents treated the vomiting?
     d. Are there associated sxs. (e.g., fever, headache, ear ache, sore throat, cough, asthma, abdominal pain, diarrhea, rash, lethargy, seizures)?
     e. If the patient is a young infant (1-3 mo) with projectile vomiting, suspect pyloric stenosis.
  2. The PE should include an assessment of the patient's vital signs, weight, and hydration. Specific areas to highlight in the exam include:
     a. HEENT: (papilledema); ears (OM); throat (pharyngitis, cervical adenopathy); fontanelle (bulging vs. sunken).
     b. Resp: cough/wheezing.

    c. Abd: pain/distention/bowel sounds/hepato-splenomegaly.

    d. GU: R/O infection, pregnancy, toxic shock syndrome.

    e. Skin: rash.

    f. Neuro: lethargy, paresthesias, seizures, focal signs.

3. Laboratory studies depend on the suspected etiology.

    a. Blood: electrolytes, NH4, glucose, SUN, medication or toxicology levels, cbc, hepatitis serologies, LFTs, bilirubin.

    b. Urine: ± metabolic screen, urine sp. gr., glucosuria, ketonuria, bilirubinuria, microscopic, ± culture.

4. Etiologies include infectious (viral-rotavirus, Norwalk virus: bacterial-enterotoxins); Toxic-metabolic (DKA, inborn error of metabolism); ↑ ICP (meningitis, Reye's syndrome, tumor); and GI obstruction (pyloric stenosis).

5. Treatment: If etiology appears to be self-limited infectious process (e.g., viral; enterotoxin), and if patient is not significantly dehydrated and can retain sufficient liquids to maintain hydration, outpatient therapy should be tried.

    a. D/C solid foods and milk

    b. For infants - Oral glucose-electrolyte solution: Frequent, small feedings x 12-24 hr. Advance to regular diet as tolerated over 24-48 hr.
    For older children - Coca-cola, Kool-Aid, Hawaiian punch; popsicles; frequent, small feedings x 12-24 hr. Advance to BRATS diet (bananas, rice, applesauce, toast, saltines) over next day. Finally, advance to regular diet.

REFERENCES

Abdominal Pain

1. Gellis S, Kagan B: *Current Pediatric Therapy*, 10. Philadel-ph-ia: WB Saunders, 1982. pp. 188-192.
2. Tunnessen W: *Signs and Symptoms in Pediatrics*. Philadel-ph-ia: JB Lippincott Co, 1983, pp. 321-9.
3. Barr R: Abdominal pain in the female adolescent. *Pediatr in Rev* 1983; 4:281-9.
4. Barbero G: Recurrent abdominal pain in childhood. *Pediatr in Rev* 1982; 4:29-34.
5. Coleman W, Levine M: Recurrent abdominal pain. *Pediatr in Rev* 1986; 8:143-51.
6. Olson A: Recurrent abodminal pain-An approach to diag-nosis and management. *Pediatr Annals* 1987; 16:834-42.
7. Lennard-Jones JE: Functional gastrointestinal disorders. *NEJM* 1983; 308:431-5.

Gastrointestinal Bleeding

1. DeAngelis C: *Pediatric Primary Care*, 3rd ed. Boston: Little,Brown, and Co., 1984. pp. 241-2.
2. Tunnessen W: *Signs and Symptoms in Pediatrics*. Philadel-phia:J.B. Lippincott Co., 1983, pp. 382-91.
3. Cox K, Ament M: Upper gastrointestinal bleeding in chil-dren and adolescents. *Pediatr* 1979; 63:408-13.
4. Rudolph A, Hoffman J: *Pediatrics*. Norwalk, Conn: Apple-ton & Lange, 1987. pp. 903-5.

Constipation

1. DeAngelis C: *Pediatric Primary Care*, 3rd ed. Boston: Little, Brown and Co., 1984. p. 229.
2. Fitzgerald J: Constipation in children. *Pediatr in Rev* 1987; 8:299-302.
3. Pettei M: Chronic constipation. *Pediatr Annals* 1987; 16:796-813.
4. Sondheimer J: Helping the child with chronic constipa-tion. *Contemp Pediatr* 1985; 1:12-28.

Diarrhea

1. Edelman R, Levine M: Acute diarrheal infections in in-fants. *Hosp Pract* 1980; 97:104.
2. Fitzgerald J: Management of the infant with persistent diarrhea. *Pediatr Infect Dis* 1985; 4:6-9.

3. Hamilton JR: Viral diarrhea: *Pediatr Annals* 1985; 14:25-50.
4. Levine J: Chronic nonspecific diarrhea. *Pediatr Annals* 1987; 16:821-9.
5. Lo C, Walker WA: Chronic protracted diarrhea of infancy - A Nutritional Disease. *Pediatr* 1983; 72:786-800.
6. Merritt R et al: Treatment of Protracted Diarrhea of Infancy. *AJDC* 1984; 138:770-4.
7. San Joaquin V, Marks M: New agents in diarrhea. *Pediatr Infect Dis* 1982; 1:53-65.
8. Walker WA: Benign chronic diarrhea of infancy. *Pediatr in Rev* 1981; 3:153-8.

Encopresis
1. DeAngelis C: *Pediatric Primary Care*, 3rd ed. Boston: Little, Brown & Co., 1984. pp. 234-6.
2. Landman G, Rappaport L: Pediatric management of severe treatment-resistant encopresis. Dev and Beha. *Pediatr* 1985; 6:349-51.
3. Levine M: The school child with encopresis. *Pediatr in Rev* 1981; 2:285-90.

Gastroesophageal Reflux
1. Berquist W, et al: Gastroesophageal reflux - associated recurrent pneumonia and chronic asthma in children. *Pediatr* 1981; 68:29-35.
2. Herbst J: Gastroesophageal reflux. *J Pediatr* 1981; 98:859-70.
3. Herbst J: Diagnosis and treatment of gastroesophageal reflux in children. *Pediatr in Rev* 1983; 5:75-79.
4. Meyers W, Herbst J: Effectiveness of positioning therapy for gastroesophageal reflux. *Pediatr* 1982; 69:768-72.
5. Rudolph A, Hoffman J: *Pediatics*. Norwalk, Conn: Appleton and Lange; 1987. pp. 906-8.

Foreign Body Ingestion
1. DeAngelis C: *Pediatric Primary Care*, 3rd ed. Boston: Little, Brown and Co., 1984. pp. 236-7.

Vomiting
1. Rudolph A, Hoffman J: *Pediatrics*. Norwalk, Conn: Appleton & Lang; 1987. pp. 902-3.

8

GENITOURINARY DISORDERS

A. Enuresis

1. Enuresis is involuntary emission of urine that occurs after a child reaches the age when bladder control is usually attained (age 4 yr).
   a. Children who have never attained bladder control are primary enuretics; those who had such control but subsequently lost it are secondary enuretics.
   b. Before age 5 yr, primary enuresis is more common; secondary enuresis is more common after 5 yr.
   c. Enuresis may be nocturnal, diurnal, or both. Diurnal enuresis in a child older than 5 yr usually is associated with an organic disorder.
2. Important historical information includes:
   a. Age of attainment of bladder control,
   b. Type of enuresis (nocturnal, diurnal),
   c. Frequency of accidents,
   d. How the child is treated after an accident,
   e. Possible precipitating events leading to enuresis ("too busy playing to go the bathroom"),
   f. Presence of other GU symptoms (dysuria, frequency, urgency, hesistancy, dribbling, itching),
   g. Presence of constipation,

      h. Amount and types of fluids ingested in an average day,

      i. Presence of psychological problems or change in the child's familial, social, or scholastic milieu,

      j. The age of sucessful toilet-training of siblings and parents,

      k. The concomitant presence of encopresis.

3. A complete PE (including neurologic) is usually normal.

      a. The blood pressure should be measured.

      b. Particular attention should be paid to the perineum to determine the presence of erythema, edema, signs of trauma, anatomic anomalies, or the presence of urethral/vaginal discharge.

      c. The abdomen should be palpated for organomegaly (bladder and kidneys), stools, and masses.

      d. A rectal exam should be done, especially noting sphincter tone.

4. A U/A and urine culture should be done on all enuretics.

Radiologic evaluation of the GU tract is necessary for children with diurnal enuresis, recalcitrant enuretics, children who constantly dribble, or those with external GU anatomic anomalies.

5. Some causes of enuresis are:

      a. Urinary tract infections (see p. 117).

      b. Ectopic ureter.

      c. Other GU organic lesions.

      d. Small bladder capacity (maturational delay in size).

      e. Ingestion of increased amounts of fluids.

      f. Ingestion of caffeine, theophylline, chocolate, diuretics.

      g. Inattention (too busy to void).

      h. Psychological problems (fear, anger, resentment, etc., especially in conjunction with a new sibling or change in the child's social, familial, or scholastic milieu).

      i. Diabetes mellitus, diabetes insipidus.
      j. Post-ictal states.
      k. Child abuse (especially sexual abuse).
      l. Perineal irritation (masturbation, trauma, infection, chemical irritation, etc.).

6. Treatment of the primary enuretic includes:
    a. Reassurance (spontaneous cure rate of 10% per yr after 5 yr of age)
    b. Bladder stretching exercise (family establishes child's baseline intake and output; child is then encouraged to force fluids and hold his urine for as long as possible each day-3 to 6 mo required),
    c. A reward system for a certain number of dry nights (goal should be attainable and dynamic),
    d. Discouraging fluid intake after dinner,
    e. Voiding before bedtime,
    f. An enuresis alarm (alarm's sounding sensitizes sleeping child to sensation of a full bladder, so that, ultimately, he awakens when his bladder is full but has not yet voided),
    g. Counseling or psychotherapy (if indicated).
    h. The use of imipramine has been widely advocated; it depresses both bladder contractions and REM sleep. However, concerns over its myocardial effects and its potential for overdosage have made it less popular; it should not be used.
    i. Secondary enuretics should have the precipitating disorder addressed and managed.

B. Dysuria, Hesitancy, Urgency, Dribbling

1. Dysuria (painful urination), hesitancy (inability to start stream), urgency (heightened pressure to void), and dribbling (passing a few drops of urine after voiding is completed) may be signs of urinary tract infection; genital infection; perineal irritation (trauma, tight clothing, harsh soaps, bubble baths or shampooing in the bath, masturbation);

sexual abuse; or emotional disorders.

2. For pertinent history, physical, and lab workup, see Section C, below, "Frequency," #2-4.

3. Treatment is directed to the underlying disorder.

C. Frequency

1. Frequency denotes a pattern of increased urination compared to one's normal pattern. There may be more frequent voiding episodes, more urine produced with each episode, or both.

2. Important historical information includes:
   a. Age of attainment of bladder control,
   b. Normal voiding pattern,
   c. Duration of new pattern,
   d. Ingestion of large amounts of fluids,
   e. Ingestion of medications or caffeine-containing products,
   f. The possibility of trauma or abuse,
   g. The presence of other GU symptoms (dysuria, hesitancy, urgency, enuresis, change in urine color or odor).

3. The PE should be complete with particular attention paid to the perineum (redness and swelling of urethra and penile discharge; redness, bruises, swelling, excoriations of the urethra, labia, clitoral areas; vaginal discharge or odor). The perianal area should be examined for excoriations and signs of trauma.

4. A urine should be microscopically examined for blood cells and bacteria; its pH and specific gravity should be assessed; the presence of glucose, protein, ketones, blood, bilirubin should be determined by dipstick.
   A culture is indicated if there is a penile or vaginal discharge; it should also be gram-stained.

5. Causes of frequency
   a. Urinary tract infection - (see p. 117)
   b. Diabetes mellitus - a positive dipstick for urinary glucose ($\pm$ ketones) necessitates a serum

glucose determination (see Ch. 5, A, "Diabetes").

c. Diabetes insipidus: failure to raise one's urine specific gravity above 1.010 even in the face of 6-12 hr of fluid deprivation necessitates a serum osmolality determination

d. Vaginitis/urethritis (see Ch. 8, L, "Vaginal Problems," "STD's").

e. Excessive fluid intake.

f. Diuretic ingestion.

g. Caffeine/theophylline ingestion.

h. Irritation of urethra/vagina (especially trauma, tight clothing, harsh soaps, bubble baths or shampooing in the bath, masturbation).

i. Emotional problems.

j. Sexual abuse.

6. Treatment of frequency is accomplished by correcting the underlying condition.

D. Hematuria

1. The presence of microscopic hematuria may be noted by dipstick in asymptomatic children during health assessment visits. Remember, a dipstick is very sensitive and may be positive in the presence of only 2-5 RBC's/HPF. When macroscopic hematuria is present, it usually is the reason for the child's visit.

2. Macroscopic hematuria may be caused by:
   a. Trauma,
   b. Tumors,
   c. Sickle cell trait,
   d. Renal stones,
   e. Hypercalcuria without stones,
   f. Hyperuricosuria,
   g. GU disorders,
   h. Benign recurrent hematuria,
   i. Alport syndrome (hereditary nephritis with nerve deafness),

      j. Glomerulonephritis (smoky, colored urine, hypertension, oliguria, edema),

      k. Hemorrhagic cystitis,

      l. Urinary tract infection,

      m. Hematospermia (in adolescent males).

3. Microscopic (or variable) hematuria may be present in the conditions listed in #2 and also in:

      a. Connective tissue disease - induced nephritis,

      b. Hemolytic-uremic syndrome,

      c. Henoch-Schönlein purpura,

      d. Leukemia,

      e. Certain malignancies,

      f. Thrombocytopenia or clotting disorders,

      g. Renal vein thrombosis,

      h. Subacute bacterial endocarditis,

      i. Hemangiomas of the GU tract,

      j. Polycystic renal disease,

      k. Urinary tract anomalies,

      l. Renal tuberculosis,

      m. Hydronephrosis,

      n. Scurvy,

      o. Mumps,

      p. Rubeola,

      q. Varicella,

      r. Malaria,

      s. Schistosomiasis,

      t. Exercise; running; boxing; wrestling,

      u. Ingestions (aspirin, anticoagulants, Elavil, lead, methicillin, phenol, sulfa drugs, and turpentine - to name a few).

4. History should elicit:

      a. The onset and duration of the hematuria,

      b. Its color (or color change) and amount,

      c. GU symptoms

      d. A history of trauma, chronic medical conditions, medication use, or ingestions,

      e. Previous GU surgery,

      f. GU disease,

      g. An antecedent sore throat (AGN),

  h. Colicky pain (stones),
  i. Allergies,
  j. Deafness in patient or other family members (Alport's syndrome),
  k. Other family members with hematuria (familial hematuria),
  l. Easy bleeding (hematologic disorders),
  m. Bloody diarrhea (HUS, HSP),
  n. Dyspnea or fatigue or change in a known murmur (SBE),
  o. Diet (scurvy),
  p. Other illnesses present concomitantly (mumps, varicella, rubeola),
  q. A travel history (malaria, schistosomiasis),
  r. Exertion.
5. A complete PE must be done. It may be normal or markedly abnormal depending on the etiology of the bleeding. The child's vital signs should be stabilized.
6. Laboratory tests are dictated by the clinical impression.
  a. Macroscopic hematuria should be evaluated with a cbc with diff, platelet count, and clotting studies; serum BUN and creatinine; electrolytes; sickle cell prep (if the child is black and his sickle status is unknown).
  b. If AGN is suspected, ESR, ANA, IgA, serum complement (C3) levels, ASO titers, and a T/C should be obtained.
  c. If SBE is suspected, an ECHO and multiple blood cultures should be obtained.
  d. When stones are suspected, a flat plate of the abdomen or ultrasound should be performed.
  e. If trauma has occurred, an IVP may localize the lesion.
7. Treatment is directed to the underlying condition.
  a. Some conditions require no specific therapy, but only reassurance (sickle cell trait, benign hematuria, Alport's syndrome).

b. Others have recurrent hematuria as part of their sign/symptoms constellation (connective tissue diseases); patients should be so warned with instructions about which symptoms require attention.

c. Surgical problems and significant trauma should be repaired.

d. Infections should be treated with the appropriate antimicrobial.

e. Malignancies and tumors are treated surgically or with chemotherapy.

f. Hematologic disorders are treated with replacement therapy when appropriate (e.g., fresh frozen plasma, whole bood, etc).

g. HSP and HUS have been discussed elsewhere.

h. AGN is treated with fluid restriction, diuretics, and antihypertensives (usually hydralazine or reserpine; may need diazoxide if malignant hypertension).

i. Hypercalcuria is treated with diuretics.

j. Hyperuricosuria is treated with allopurinol.

E. Hernia

1. An inguinal hernia is the protrusion of abdominal structures into the scrotum or inguinal region. This is due to the persistence of a peritoneal sac, the processus vaginalis, which normally becomes fibrotic late in gestation.

   a. Hernias may occur in both males and females, since the processus vaginalis precedes both the testis in its descent into the inguinal canal and scrotum, and the round ligament in its descent into the canal and labia.

   b. The male-to-female ratio of hernias is 5-6:1; in a female bilateral inguinal hernias with palpable contents (? gonads) should prompt suspicion of an endocrine or genetic problem.

   c. In addition, most (85-90%) hernias are unilateral; the right side predominates. The size is variable.

2. Important historical information includes duration and location of the mass, whether it changes in size (especially if it becomes larger on exertion or crying), and the events that precipitate size changes.

   If incarceration of the hernia is suspected, a history of vomiting, scant stooling, melena, irritability, and abdominal distension should be sought.

3. On PE, a mass may be palpated in the scrotum or labia; this mass may be more easily appreciated if the child is crying or straining (increased intra-abdominal pressure).

   a. The hernia usually does not transilluminate, and bowel sounds are usually heard on auscultation.

   b. Most hernias are manually reducible by the examiner, because the contents of the processus ordinarily slide in and out of the abdominal cavity. However, if the neck of the sac closes over the herniated abdominal contents, the hernia may not be reducible (incarcerated hernia).

   c. If the hernia is tender, swollen, and warm, it is strangulated. Vascular compromise may lead to bowel gangrene.

4. Treatment is surgical.

   a. The hernia sac (patent processus vaginalis) is closed at the inguinal ring. Because there is a significant incidence of contralateral hernia sacs, bilateral exploration may be done. Surgical repair should be performed as soon as possible after the hernia is discovered.

   b. An incarcerated hernia may be manually reduced under sedation. If successful, a herniorrhaphy should be performed within 1-2 days; if unsuccessful, immediate surgery is necessary.

F. **Hydrocele**

1. A hydrocoele is a collection of peritoneal fluid in the scrotum. An accompanying hernia may or may

not be present. If the size of the hydrocele varies over time, suspect an open tunica vaginalis (indirect hernia). If the hydrocoele's size is constant, the tunica vaginalis is closed.

2. Important historical information includes duration of scrotal swelling and whether the size of the swelling varies both during rest and during times of emotional unrest (crying, fear).

3. On PE, the hydrocele feels ovoid or round, smooth, and non-tender. Scrotal skin is normal.
   A hydrocele may be differentiated from a hernia in several ways. A hydrocele cannot be reduced; a hernia usually can. A hydrocele is translucent when transilluminated, while a hernia is not. Finally, auscultation of the scrotum for bowel sounds is unsuccessful when a hydrocele is present and is usually successful (except when the loop of bowel is strangulated) when there is a hernia.

4. A hydrocele that is constant in size usually indicates that no hernia is present; no treatment is necessary as the fluid gradually reabsorbs. If the hydrocele is accompanied by a hernia, treatment is as discussed in the previous section, "Hernia."

G. Proteinuria

1. When protein is present in the urine, its concentration may be estimated by a dipstick impregnated with tetrabromphenol (trace - 10 mg/100 cc; 1+ = 30 mg/100cc; 2+ = 100 mg/100 cc; 3+ = 300 mg/100 cc; 4+ = 1000 mg/100 cc).
   a. Some degree of proteinuria is found in 5-15% of routine urinalyses; a falsely positive dipstick for proteinuria may occur if the urine's pH is basic.
   b. Total daily protein excretion should be <100 mg.

2. Transient proteinuria
   a. May be due to fever, epinephrine, cold exposure, blood transfusions, burns, and exercise.
   b. Orthostatic proteinuria is present in the upright position but absent in the supine (diagnosed by

obtaining a urine sample <u>before</u> the child gets out of bed and another <u>after</u> he has been up for several hours or his last void before he goes to bed). Orthostatic proteinuria is benign; it rarely is more than 1gm of protein spilled per day.

3. Other causes of proteinuria include analgesic abuse, hypokalemia, vitamin D intoxication, nephritis, and nephrosis.

4. When proteinuria is discovered as an incidental finding during a health assessment visit, the history and physical are usually unrevealing as to its etiology.

   a. Questions about GU symptoms, edema and its location, exercise and any weight gain, antecedent sore throat (especially if hematuria is also present), and family members with proteinuria should be asked.

   b. The PE should determine if the kidneys can be palpated (i.e., enlargement), if there is edema, or if the perineum is abnormal in any way.

   c. The urine should be examined microscopically for evidence of infection, and a culture is indicated.

5. If the child has 1+ protein or more, a second urine sample (on another day) should be obtained. If this sample is also positive, orthostatic and exercise-induced proteinuria should be ruled out. A urine culture should also be obtained.

   a. If the evaluation is unrevealing and proteinuria (2+ or greater) continues, a 24-h urine for protein should be obtained.

   b. Also indicated are serum proteins (including albumin), creatinine, BUN, cholesterol, complement (C_3) and ASO titers (<u>especially</u> if hematuria is present, as the proteinuria may be secondary to post-streptococcal nephritis).

   c. A renal biopsy may eventually need to be obtained to secure a diagnosis.

H. Testicular Swelling/Pain

1. The normal prepubertal testis is 1 x 2 cm in size; by adulthood, the testis measures 2.5-3.0 x 4.0-4.5 cm. When there is testicular enlargement or pain, several diagnoses must be considered.

   a. Testicular Torsion (torsion of the spermatic core): This is an emergency, as continued torsion results in gangrene of the testis. The child presents with sudden, unilateral testicular pain; his testis is swollen and tender and the overlying scrotal skin is red and warm. Lifting the testis gently does not relieve the pain (Prehn's sign). He may have a fever and be vomiting. Lack of urinary symtoms is the rule and urinalysis is normal. If the diagnosis is in doubt, a technetium-99 pertechnetate scan will confirm it. However, since the risk of gangrene is high, there should be no delay in definitive treatment, which is surgery. Orchiectomy is usually necessary if the torsion has been present > 24 hr.

   b. Epididymitis (inflammation of the epididymis). The child presents with unilateral testicular pain; the epididymis is swollen and tender, and the testis may also be involved ("Orchitis" - see below). Scrotal skin is red on the affected side. Unlike testicular torsion, lifting the scrotum does bring pain diminution. He may have a fever, chills, dysuria/frequency. A microscopic urine exam may demonstrate bacteria and pyuria; <u>Escherichia coli</u> is the common infecting agent in prepubertal boys. In postpubertal, sexually active boys (especially those with a penile discharge), gonorrhea and chlamydia must be considered; gram stain and culture the discharge.
   Treatment consists of immediate antibiotic use (initially ampicillin, final choice based on the culture and sensitivity results of urine or urethral discharge); sitz baths tid-qid; and scrotal

support. If an STD is diagnosed, sexual partners must be treated also.

c. Orchitis (inflammation of the testis): The prepubertal child presents with fever, chills, scrotal swelling, and pain. The postpubertal boy presents similarly, and he also may have urinary symptoms and a penile discharge (usually gonorrhea). In both age groups, elevating the scrotum will diminish the pain. Urine and penile discharge should be appropriately stained, examined microscopically, and cultured. The usual cause of orchitis in a prepubertal child is mumps (with or without parotid swelling); serum amylase will be elevated.

Treatment for the self-limited (7-14 days) mumps orchitis consists of sitz baths and scrotal support. Treatment for orchitis due to gonorrhea includes sitz baths, scrotal support, and antibiotic therapy. (See Ch. 19, B, "Gonorrhea.")

d. Testicular Trauma: Usually due to a direct blow to the scrotum, which then is tender, bruised, and swollen. Physical examination may be extremely painful for the child. A urine sample should be examined for the presence of hematuria (urethral, renal trauma).

Treatment consists of ice packs to the area (24-48 h followed by sitz baths), elevation of the scrotum, or scrotal support.

e. Tumor.

I. Undescended Testis

1. A testis may be considered "undescended" if (a) it rides high in the scrotum or (2) it is not palpable (testicular agenesis or ectopic testis).

   a. A rectractile testis is one that is normally descended but is intermittently retracted due to the action of the cremasteric muscle.

   b. Undescended testes may be unilateral or bilateral. In the patient with bilateral undescended

testes, serum FSH and LH levels should be done to R/O anorchidism.
c. The condition is common in neonates; if spontaneous descent is to occur, it will do so by 9-12 mo of age.
2. A retractile testis may be brought back into the scrotum manually, or it may descend spontaneously when the child is relaxed, squats, or is bathing in warm water. Retractile testes require no therapy.
3. Although administration of human chorionic gonadotropin over several wk may medically reposition bilaterally undescended testes, most children require surgery (orchiopexy with concomitant inguinal herniorrhaphy) before age 5 yr to preserve fertility.

J. Urethritis

1. Characterized by erythema of the urethra and dysuria; may or may not have purulent discharge.
2. Etiology includes:
   a. Purulent urethritis: gonorrhea most common. <u>Staphyloccus aureus</u>, streptococci, enteric organisms also occur.
   b. Nonpurulent urethritis: gonorrhea; <u>Chlamydia trachomatis; Ureaplasma urealyticum; Trichomonas;</u> mycoplasmas.
   c. Noninfectious causes: chemical (soaps, bubble baths, powders), traumatic, physical irritation to urethra (masturbation); and Reiter's syndrome (urethritis, arthritis, and conjunctivitis; etiology unknown).
3. Evaluation
   a. Do gram stain; send culture for GC and routine bacteria. <u>Trichomonas</u> and <u>Chlamydia</u> require special media.
   b. Wet saline prep (look for Trichomonas).
   c. Treatment
      1) GC - see Ch. 19, "Sexually Transmitted Diseases."

2) Non-gonococcal (e.g., <u>Chlamydia</u> most common) - tetracycline 500 mg qid x 14 d (Erythromycin is alternate Rx during pregnancy).

3) If noninfectious - remove irritating factor.

K. Urinary Tract Infections

1. Symptoms vary and can be nonspecific (especially in younger children).
   a. Some associated symptoms include dysuria, frequency, urgency, enuresis.
   b. Nonspecific symptoms include vomiting, diarrhea, fever, lethargy, irritability, failure to thrive, abdominal pain.
   c. Dysuria and frequency may also be associated with urethritis (check for vaginal infection, H/O tight underwear, bubble baths, trauma); consider GC, chlamydial, or other STDs.
   d. Some UTIs are asymptomatic. Both symptomatic and asymptomatic UTIs may lead to renal compromise.
2. The PE is frequently normal, but emphasis should be placed on the abdominal exam (masses, suprapubic tenderness), CVA area (tenderness), and perineum (redness, excoriations, discharge). The blood pressure should be checked.
3. Diagnosis varies with method of obtaining specimen.
   a. Urine culture:
      1) Clean catch urine: >100,000 col/cc of single organism x 2 consecutive specimens.
      2) Catheterized urine: >100 col/cc of single organism x 1 specimen.
      3) Suprapubic urine: growth of any organism.
      NOTE: The standard of >100,000 col of any organism per cc of midstream urine as diagnostic of a UTI is based on studies of adult females. This standard may not be valid for pediatric patients, and strict adherence to this standard may result in

missed diagnoses of UTI in symptomatic patients. Make certain patient or parent really knows how to obtain "clean catch." The child's urethral meatus and surrounding area are cleaned. He then begins to void. After his stream has started, the midstream specimen is collected.

b. Urine analysis: Examination of the urine is valuable but <u>not</u> sufficient to dx UTI. A negative analysis does not R/O a UTI. A patient may or may not have any of the following on analysis:

1) Pyuria: if >10 WBCs/hpf spun specimen, then positive culture rate is >40%.
2) Hematuria.
3) Bacteriuria: >1 organism/hpf on unstained, unspun urine associated with 10^5 col/cc (100,000 col/cc).
4) Granular casts: associated with pyelonephritis.
5) Also check for protein, sugar, pH, concentration.

4. Etiologies: <u>E. coli</u> most frequent organism. Other common pathogens include <u>Enterobacter, Klebsiella, Proteus species</u>, and <u>Enterococcus</u>. <u>S. aureus</u> and <u>Pseudomonas</u> are more likely to be recovered after antimicrobial therapy or instrumentation.

5. Treatment

a. Sulfisoxazole (Gantrisin) 150 mg/kg/day divided qid (max 6 gm/d) x 14d or ampicillin 100 mg/kg/ day divided qid x 14 d (max 2 gm/d).

b. Don't start treatment until you have obtained at least 2 clean catch urines or one suprapubic or catheter specimen (to avoid problems with equivocal urine culture results).

c. In infants <8 weeks, sepsis is frequently associated with UTI. Workup appropriately. Rx with IV ampicillin and gentamicin in hospital.

6. Suggested follow-up

a. Return in 48 hr for repeat U/A and culture to document sterile urine and clinical improvement. This will help to identify resistant organisms.

      b. Return 1-3 wk after antibiotics discontinued for U/A and culture.

      c. Do subsequent follow-up cultures every 1-3 mo until patient has remained free of infection for 1 yr, then yearly.

  7. Recurrences

      a. Recurrence in 25% of males and 30-80% of females within the first yr. Often asymptomatic.

      b. If necessary, consider prophylaxis with trimethoprim - sulfamethoxazole, or nitrofurantoin for 6 mo to one yr.

      c. Avoid urologic procedures such as urethral dilation.

  8. Further evaluation

      a. The indications for obtaining a renal US (formerly IVP) and VCUG are debatable.

      b. The official recommendation of the American Academy of Pediatrics is that a radiologic workup should be performed on all children (male and female) after one documented UTI.

      c. Others recommend that in females >12 mo, an IVP and VCUG be done only after a second UTI. (This radiologic evaluation should be scheduled <u>after</u> treating infection, because 50% of children will have vesicoureteral reflux <u>during</u> acute infection period.)

      d. Children <4 yrs of age and males are more likely to have structural problems (e.g. vesicoureteral reflux or ureteral obstruction). Renal scarring (usually secondary to reflux or obstruction) is most likely to occur in pre-school children.

L. Vaginal Problems

  1. <u>Vulvovaginitis & Vaginitis:</u> May occur at any age.

      a. Symptoms include itching, discharge, dysuria (if urethritis also present), erythema/edema of vulva or vagina.

      b. Etiology may be noninfectious or infectious.

   1) Noninfectious: trauma, foreign body (mal-
      odorous, often bloody discharge), chemical
      irritant or allergen (OTC douches, powders,
      bubble bath), masturbation, tumor. Nylon
      panties prevent evaporation of normal mois-
      ture; their use may promote vaginitis.
   2) Infectious:
      a) Nonspecific: Bacterial overgrowth of enter-
         ic organisms secondary to poor perineal
         hygiene; Gardnerella vaginalis.
      b) Specific: gonorrhea, monilia, trichomonas,
         B-hemolytic strep, chlamydia, pinworms;
         herpes simplex virus.
   c. Evaluation:
      1) Examine external genitalia for scratches, tears,
         redness, ulcers, discharge, swelling. Vaginos-
         copy may be performed in prepubertal fe-
         male using veterinary otoscopy speculum.
         GYN consult may be needed.
      2) Culture indicated if clinical symptoms are
         present with or without discharge, ulcera-
         tions (in young female, may need to obtain
         culture using medicine dropper filled with
         nonbacteriostatic saline: inject saline and
         aspirate for vaginal culture). Evaluate vagi-
         nal specimen by wet saline mount
         (Trichomonas), KOH prep (Monilia), and
         Gram stain (intracellular gram negative
         diplococci). Do both a GC and routine cul-
         ture.
      3) Foreign bodies are characteristically associat-
         ed with foul-smelling discharges. FBs may
         be palpable by digital rectal exam in a prepu-
         bertal female, but the most common FB (toi-
         let paper) usually is not palpable. One can
         do a vaginal flush using normal saline intro-
         duced into the vagina via an infant feeding
         tube connected to a 30 cc syringe. Do not
         exert excess force to the plunger of the

syringe (possibility of retrograde flow up cervix). Examination under anesthesia might be necessary.

d. Agent-specific treatment

    1) For nonspecific vaginitis:

        a) Remove irritating factor (FB, douche, bubble bath, etc.).

        b) Parents should instruct child on proper wiping technique (front to back, not back to front).

        c) Warm sitz baths tid.

        d) Loose fitting white cotton panties.

        e) Reassure parents about normalcy of masturbation.

        f) For cases resistant to the above therapy: Reassess: Make sure you have done adequate cultures and ruled out abuse, FBs, anatomic defects, etc.

    2) <u>Monilia</u>:

        a) Intense pruritus, thick curdy discharge, dysuria.

        b) Predisposing factors: oral contraceptives, antibiotics, diabetes. Very common in postpubertal females.

        c) Diagnosis by KOH prep. Sometimes you can see darkly stained hyphae on gram stain. KOH may miss 50% of culture positive specimens.

        d) Treatment

            (1) Monistat cream intravaginally q hs x 1-2 wk. Wear minipad to keep cream from coming out during the day.

            (2) Clotrimazole 100 mg intravaginal tablets, 1 hs x 1-2 wk.

    3) <u>Trichomonas</u>

        a) Greenish-yellow discharge, foul odor, pruritus, dyspareunia.

        b) Diagnosis by saline wet mount.

        c) Treatment

(1) Metronidazole (Flagyl) - if not pregnant, 2 gm po in single dose (preferred); 250 mg tid x 7 days for failure.

(2) Clotrimazole 100 mg, intravaginally hs, x 7 d if pregnant. Treat the partner to prevent reinfection.

4) <u>Gardnerella vaginalis</u> (formerly <u>Hemophilus vaginalis</u>)

  a) Gray frothy discharge, fishy odor, pruritus not prominent.

  b) Diagnosis by presence of "clue cells" (epithelial cells covered with bacteria) and absence of trichomonas and monilia.

  c) Treatment

    (1) Ampicillin 500 mg qid x 10 d

      or

      Tetracycline 500 mg qid x 10 d (if patient is not pregnant).

      Not all cases will respond to this regimen.

      Often a good idea to treat concomitantly with Nystastin cream to avoid superinfection with <u>Monilia</u>.

    (2) Metronidazole (Flagyl) 500 mg bid x 7 d. Effective therapy, but uncertainty about carcinogenicity remains.

    (3) Treat the partner if antibiotics used.

5) Group A beta-hemolytic strep: Oral penicillin in same dosage as for strep pharyngitis.

6) Treatment for GC and HSV included in Ch. 19 "Sexually Transmitted Diseases."

2. Vaginal Bleeding

  a. Vaginal bleeding may be due to trauma (straddle injury, inanimate object penetration, sexual abuse), menstruation, spotting during early pregnancy, abortion, ingestion of birth control pills, use (improper) of birth control pills, maternal estrogen effect (neonates who may

also have breast enlargement), vaginal infections, FBs, tumors.
b. Obtain history of duration and amount of vaginal bleeding, precipitating events, whether bleeding waxes and wanes, history of trauma, abuse, FB, birth control pill ingestion, other GU symptoms.
c. Examine perineum carefully.
   1) Look for contusions, lacerations of labia, vagina, and urethra.
   2) Check hymenal integrity (virginal prepubertal hymen < 1 cm).
   3) Is bleeding brisk from vagina or slow and sporadic?
   4) Are there any masses present?
   5) If the patient is sexually active or has had previous pelvic exams, do a pelvic to determine if blood is coming from the cervical os (if os is open), if cervix is eroded, or if a FB is present. Do a bimanual and rectal exam to check for masses and FBs.
   6) If the child is prepubertal, she may require sedation for an adequate inspection of her vagina and cervix. Vaginoscopy may be performed by using a veterinary otoscope speculum. A rectal exam should be done to check for masses or a FB.
d. If vaginal bleeding is profuse, a Hct should be checked.
   1) Clotting studies may be indicated if there are petechiae, purpura, or other bleeding sites.
   2) If there is evidence of an infection, appropriate culturing should be done in addition to a gram stain of the discharge or exudate.
   3) If the girl is sexually active, a urine/serum pregnancy test should be obtained.
e. Treatment is directed toward the underlying condition.

1) The trauma victim may require surgical repair under sedation or anesthesia by a gynecologist.
2) Foreign bodies should be removed and the vagina flushed with normal saline.
3) Vaginal/cervical infections should be appropriately treated (See "Ch. 19 "Sexually Transmitted Diseases").
4) The proper strength of oral contraceptives should be chosen and their proper administration encouraged.
5) The mothers of neonates with vaginal bleeding should be reassured . Such bleeding should cease by 10 days of age.

3. Labial Adhesions
   a. Labial adhesions are epithelial agglutinations that cover the hymen and sometimes the urethral meatus. They are caused by superficial inflammation of the labia minora and usually occur in prepubertal girls. Adhesions may be complete or partial. Girls with adhesions should be observed while voiding to ensure an adequate stream.
   b. Adhesions will disappear by puberty when estrogen levels rise.
   c. If the girl has dysuria, a urinary tract infection, or chronically poor hygiene, an estrogen cream may be applied each night for 7-14 d to simulate the estrogen effect that will occur at puberty. Estrogen cream should not be used for more than 14 d, as such use may promote signs of precocious puberty.
   d. Adhesions should never be cut or manually broken, since they will recur.

REFERENCE

Enuresis
1. DeAngelis C: *Pediatric Primary Care*, 3rd ed. Boston: Little, Brown & Co., 1984. pp. 411-14.
2. Foxman B, Valdez RB, Brook R: Childhood enuresis - Prevalence, perceived impact and prescribed treatments. *Pediatr* 1986; 77:482-7.
3. Marshall F: Urinary incontinence in children. *Pediatr in Rev;* 1984; 5:209-15.
4. Smith L: Nocturnal Enuresis. *Pediatr in Rev* 1980; 2:183-6.
5. Tunnessen W: *Signs and Symptoms in Pediatrics*. Philadelphia; JB Lippincott Co., 1983; pp. 411-14.

Hematuria
1. DeAngelis C: *Pediatric Primary Care*, 3rd ed. Boston: Little, Brown & Co., 1984. p. 262.
2. Kallen R: What's causing hematuria? Contemp *Pediatr* 1986; 2:55-71.
3. Kaplan M: Hematuria in childhood. *Pediatr in Rev* 1983; 5:99-105.
4. Maurer H (ed): *Pediatrics*. New York: Churchill Living stone, 1983. p. 468-9.
5. Tunnessen W: *Signs and Symptoms in Pediatrics*. Philadelphia: JB Lippincott Co., 1983. pp. 400-6.
6. West C: Asymptomatic hematuria and proteinuria in children. *J Pediatr* 1976; 89:173-82.

Hernia/Hydrocele
1. Rudolph A, Hoffman J: *Pediatrics*. Norwalk, Conn: Appleton & Lange; 1987. pp. 953-4.

Proteinuria
1. Feld L, et al: Evaluation of the child with asymptomatic proteinuria. *Pediatr in Rev* 1984; 5:248-54.
2. Maurer H (ed). *Pediatrics*. New York: Churchill Livingstone, 1983. pp. 468-9.
3. Vehaskari VM, Rapola J: Isolated proteinuria - Analysis of a school-age population. J *Pediatr* 1982; 101:661-8.
4. West C: Asymptomatic hematuria and proteinuria in children. *J Pediatr* 1976; 89:173-82.

Testicular Swelling/Pain
1. DeAngelis C: *Pediatric Primary Care*, 3rd Ed. Boston: Little, Brown & Co., 1984. pp. 267-8.
2. Likitnukul S, et al: Epididymitis in children and adolescents. *AJDC* 1987; 141:41-4.
3. Sharer W: Acute scrotal pathology. *Surg Clinics of N. Amer* 1982; 62:955-70.
4. Staller M, et al: Spermatic cord torsion - Diagnostic limitations. *Pediatr* 1985; 76:929-33.
5. Stillwell T, Kramer S: Intermittent testicular torsion. *Pediatr* 1986; 77:908-11.

Undescended Testis
1. Allen T: Cryptorchidism. *Pediatr in Rev* 1984; 5:317-9.
2. DeAngelis C: *Pediatric Primary Care*, 3rd ed. Boston: LIttle, Brown, & Co., 1984, pp. 257-8.
3. Koyle M et al: The undescended testis. *Pediatr Annals* 1988; 17:39-46.

Urethritis
1. Rosenfeld W, Litman N: Urogenital tract infections in Male Adolescents. *Pediatr in Rev* 1983; 4:257-65.

Urinary Tract Infections
1. Durbin W, Peter G: Management of urinary tract infections in infants and children. *Pediatr Infect Dis* 1984; 3:564-74.
2. Ginsburg C, McCracken G: Urinary tract infections in young infants. *Pediatr* 1982; 69:409-12.
3. McCracken G: Diagnosis and Management of Acute Urinary Tract Infections in Infants and Children. *Pediatr Infect Dis* 1987; 6:107-12.

Vaginitis
1. Altchek A: Recognizing and controlling vulvovaginitis in children. *Contemp Pediatr* 1985; 2:59-70.
2. Arsenault P, Oerbie A: Vulvovaginitis in the pre-adolescent girl. *Pediatr Annals* 1986; 15:557-85.
3. DeAngelis C: *Pediatric Primary Care*, 3rd ed. Boston: Little, Brown & Co., 1984. pp. 507-11.
4. Emans SJ: Vulvovaginitis in the child and adolescent. *Pediatr in Rev* 1986; 8:12-19.

5. Moffett H: *Pediatric Infectious Diseases*, 2nd ed. 1981. pp. 360-9.
6. Paradise J, Willis E: Probability of vaginal foreign body in girls with genital complaints. *AJDC* 1985; 139:472-6.
7. Tunnessen W: *Signs and Symptoms in Pediatrics*. Philadelphia: JB Lippincott Co., 1983, pp. 432-5.

Vaginal Bleeding
1. Anderson M et al: Abnormal vaginal bleeding in adolescents. *Pediatr Annals* 1986; 15:697-707.
2. DeAngelis C: *Pediatric Primary Care*, 3rd ed. Boston: Little, Brown & Co., 1984; pp. 505:7.

Labial Adhesions
1. DeAngelis C: *Pediatric Primary Care*, 3rd ed. Boston: LIttle, Brown & Co., 1984, p. 264.
2. Williams T, et al: Vulvar disorders in the prepubertal female. *Pediatr Annals* 1986; 15:588-605.

9

HEMATOLOGY

A. Anemia:

Only a sign of a disease or blood loss. Must determine etiology.

1. Normal values and indices: See *Harriet Lane Handbook.* In Blacks, Hgb may run 0.5 gm% lower.

2. Nadir "physiologic anemia" of term infant at 8-12 wk. Hct should not be <30%. After this nadir, Hct should be >32% and MCV >77u³.

3. History
   a. Any known blood loss (stool, urine, nosebleeds, perinatal problems etc.)?
   b. Source of dietary Fe (formula, meats, cereals, vitamins + Fe)?
   c. H/O excess whole milk intake (>32 oz/d)?
   d. H/O pica (R/O Pb poisoning)?
   e. H/O prior anemia?
   f. FHx - ethnic/racial background.
   g. Hemoglobinopathy/gallstones/anemia/splenectomy?
   h. Is the pt taking any medications that may depress bone marrow or cause hemolysis?
   i. H/O malaise, fatigue, palpitations?

4. Exam: Look for pallor, tachycardia, petechiae, purpura, icterus, lymphadenopathy, hepatosplenomegaly, +stool guaiac, hematuria.

5. Hematology Lab: cbc with indices, reticulocyte count, peripheral blood smear (most important). More extensive workup (Pb level/FEP, hemoglobin-electrophoresis, hemoccult of the stool, G6PD, Coomb's test, haptoglobin, etc.) as indicated in selected patients.

6. Iron Deficiency Anemia
   a. Most common etiology of anemia age 6 mo to 3 yr, usually on nutritional basis. If Fe deficiency after 3 yrs, think of blood loss.
   b. Smear: RBCs will be hypochromic, microcytic; low MCV and/or MCHC: low reticulocyte count; low serum ferritin; FEP moderately elevated.
   c. Treatment of Iron Deficiency Anemia
      1) Correct basic problem: dietary, bleeding sources, etc.
      2) Elemental iron (3 mg/kg/day divided tid with meals; 2-3 mo duration will adequately replete Fe stores (e.g., Fer-in-sol drops=25 mg Fe/cc; check *Harriet Lane Handbook* for other preparations).
      3) Check 7-10 days after initiation of iron Rx- should see elevated reticulocyte count; by 4 wk, Hct should be normal;smear has two populations of RBCs (normal and Fe-deficient).
   d. Failure to Correct Presumed Iron Deficiency Anemia
      1) Poor compliance: did patient get Fe? Teeth staining, dark stools indicate Fe given. Ask parents to bring medication with them or inquire how much Fe is left in bottle.
      2) Improper administration: If administered with milk or other products high in phosphorus content, Fe may not be well absorbed.
      3) Malabsorption: malabsorption of Fe may be present in as many as 20% of Fe-deficient patients who do not respond to iron.

4) Ongoing blood losses; check stool for blood.
5) Incorrect diagnosis
   a) Lead poisoning, thalassemia, and chronic infection have hypochromic anemia also
   b) Check FEP (should be "↑ in plumbism)
   c) Check parents' indices and Hcts for thalassemia
6) Inability to utilize Fe: in the presence of concomitant lead poisoning or certain chronic disease states (especially those associated with inflammation), Fe may be absorbed but not incorporated into hemoglobin.

	MCV	RBC	RBC Distribution Width	Morphologic Anemia	Abnormalities	FEP mv µg/100 cc	Hg B Electrophoresis
Iron deficiency				+	1+	30-200	Normal
Lead poisoning	or normal	or normal		+	1-2+	>200	Normal
β- Thalassemia trait		or normal	Normal	±	2+	<90	Hb A$_2$
α Thalassemia trait		or normal	Normal	±	2+	<90	Normal

α Thalassemia trait—predominant in Orientals, blacks and Mediterraneans.
β Thalassemia Trait—mainly blacks and Mediterraneans.
Pb poisoning—peak age 6 mo-4 yrs.

B. Hemophilia

The most common inherited bleeding disorders are factor VIII deficiency (Hemophilia A), factor IX deficiency (Hemophilia B), and von Willebrand's disease (pseudohemophilia). Patients will present with bleeding episodes or following trauma that may result in hemorrhage. ER treatment includes factor replacement therapy.

1. Replacement therapy for factor VIII deficiency is cryoprecipitate or factor VIII concentrates.
2. For factor IX deficiency, replacement therapy is factor IX concentrates.
3. For von Willebrand's disease, the product of choice is cryoprecipitate or fresh frozen plasma.
4. Calculate factor level according to the type of hemorrhage and/or trauma. See *Harriet Lane Handbook*.

5. Calculation of number of units of factor VIII or factor IX necessary to achieve a specific level - See *Harriet Lane Handbook*.

WARNING: All patients with hemophilia should be considered potential hepatitis B surface antigen and HIV carriers. Gloves should be worn when drawing blood and administering replacement therapy.

C. Sickle Cell Disease

1. Vaso-occlusive crisis: infarction of bone, soft tissue, and viscera may occur as a result of intravascular sickling and vessel occlusion.

a. Bone and/or bone marrow infarction: child presents with bony pain, ± erythema, ± localized tenderness of one or more bones or joints, ± fever.

1) Always need to consider possibility of osteomyelitis or septic arthritis.

2) In general, bone infarction is much more common, and is less likely to be associated with <u>high</u> fever (>39°C), leukocytosis greater than 30,000, and systemic toxicity.

b. Pulmonary infarction: often difficult to distinguish from pneumonia on the basis of physical findings and noninvasive lab tests. Therefore, these two disorders fall under heading of "acute chest syndrome."

1) Signs and symptoms include tachypnea, rales, decreased breath sounds, dyspnea, chest pain, and abdominal pain. Some patients present initially with just abdominal pain.

2) CXR findings may be similar for both disorders.

3) All patients with chest syndrome (by physical exam and/or CXR) should have arterial PO_2 determinations.

4) Most often the patient is treated as though he has pneumonia, i.e., antibiotics, hydration, oxygen.

        5) If arterial PO_2 cannot be increased above 80 with mask O_2, then transfusion or exchange transfusion (sickle negative blood) may be indicated.

   c. Occlusion of mesenteric vessels: patient with an abdominal crisis will often present with an ileus and rebound tenderness mimicking an acute abdomen, i.e., appendicitis. The pain may be familiar to the patient and readily recognized as "crisis pain." Since painful crises are much more common than an acute surgical abdomen, a period of careful observation of clinical response to fluid therapy and analgesics is warranted in most cases.

2. Treatment of Painful Crisis
   a. Differentiation of vaso-occlusive crises from other disorders as discussed above.
   b. I.V. hydration: may start with a bolus of normal saline (20cc/kg), then fluids at 1.5 times maintenance.
      NOTE: Urine specific gravity is not helpful because of the inability of SS patients to concentrate their urine.
   c. Analgesia: acetaminophen alone, acetaminophen with codeine, or Demerol. The choice of analgesic may be aided by familiarity with the patient's previous crises. Demerol should <u>not</u> be routinely used for vaso-occlusive crisis unless acetaminophen and codeine are ineffective.
   d. Hospital admission if continuing need for parenteral analgesic therapy or if fluid intake is inadequate.

3. Presentation with fever: because of splenic dysfunction and immunologic deficiencies, patients with SS disease are susceptible to overwhelming bacterial infections, i.e., meningitis, sepsis, pneumonia, septic arthritis, osteomyelitis.
   a. May be difficult to distinguish between serious bacterial infections, self-limited viral disorders,

and vaso-occlusive crisis in a patient with fever without an obvious source.

1) Children under 4 yr of age are most susceptible to overwhelming sepsis, but older children may also be at risk.

2) Sepsis often presents as high fever with no apparent source and is not necessarily associated with a vaso-occlusive crisis.

b. Work-up: consider cbc, blood cultures, CXR, and LP. Febrile children with SS disease are generally treated as if they have bacterial infections, usually on an inpatient basis. All children with SS disease less than 4 yr old with fever and no source should be considered as potentially septic.

D. Lead Poisoning

1. a. Children with elevated lead (Pb) levels may be asymptomatic if the level is low.

   b. Mild to moderate Pb poisoning is associated with such non-specific symptoms as learning/behavior problems, fatigue, malaise, anorexia, irritability, insomnia, headache, abdominal pain, and pallor.

   c. Severe Pb poisoning is associated with clumsiness, ataxia, paresis, sensorium changes, encephalopathy with or without convulsions, optic nerve edema, splitting of cranial sutures, hypertension, bradycardia, abdominal colic, constipation, and intractable vomiting.

2. Lead is ubiquitous. It is not found just in delapidated houses with peeling paint, but is also heavily concentrated in the air and soil near highways (burning of leaded gasoline). This means that many children are exposed to high Pb levels in their environment.

3. Lead inhibits HGB production by its effects on porphyrin synthesis and iron incorporation into the porphyrin ring. One of the earliest signs of Pb

intoxication is the elevation of free erythrocyte protoporphyrin (FEP), a sensitive measure of heme synthesis.

4. To prevent the deleterious sequelae of Pb poisoning, routine Pb screening of children between the ages of 9 mo and 6 yr is recommended. Capillary samples may be used for screening, but to verify a diagnosis of Pb intoxication or to assess ongoing treatment, a venous sample should be obtained to determine the Pb and EP levels.

5. EP is measured in two ways: (a) direct fluorescence in intact red cells. EP is present as zinc protoporphyrin (ZnPP) and is measured by a hemofluorometer, and (b) extraction by acid from red cells (ET). EP levels detected as ZnPP are lower than those detected as ET. The CDC classification of Pb poisoning takes these two determination methods into account.

Class Ia: Pb $\leq$ 24 ug/dl and EP $\leq$ 174 (ZnPP) or $\leq$ 249 (ET) ug/dl

Class Ib: Pb 25-49 ug/dl and EP $\leq$ 34 ug/dl (ZnPP or ET)

Class II: Children at moderate risk-
Pb 25-49 ug/dl and EP 35-74 ug/dl (ZnPP)or 35-109 ug/dl (ET)

Class III: Children at high risk-
Pb 25-49 ug/dl and EP $\geq$ 75 ug/dl (ZnPP) or $\geq$110 ug/dl (ET)
or Pb 50-69 ug/dl and EP 35-174 (ZnPP) or 35-249 (ET)

Class IV: Children at urgent risk-
Pb 50-69 ug/dl and EP $\geq$ 175 (ZnPP) or $\geq$ 250 ug/dl (ET)
or Pb $\geq$ 70 ug/dl and EP $\geq$ 75 (ZnPP) or $\geq$ 110 ug/dl (ET)

6. In interpreting the results of screening tests, younger children ($\leq$ 3 yr) should be given priority over older ones and children whose EP and Pb

levels fall into the upper ranges of a class should have priority over those whose levels are in the lower ranges.

   a. Pb and EP values obtained on screening should be verified, with at least one venipuncture sampling.
   b. If the Pb is normal and the EP is elevated, a CBC and tests for iron deficiency should be obtained.
   c. If the Pb is elevated, depending on its level, radiographs of the abdomen and long bones (to detect Pb lines), an LP, and a provocation test (Ca Na2 EDTA Mobilization test) should be considered.

7. Management depends on the child's risk status. However, all children at risk need nutritional counseling and reduction of Pb intake. Their homes must be investigated for undue Pb burden; if found, it must be removed before the home can be considered safe.

   a. Class IV patients require immediate chelation therapy and weekly Pb/EP determinations until their decline or stabilization is documented, at which time determinations may be performed monthly.
   b. Class III children may require chelation therapy (if their provocation tests are positive) and monthly Pb/EP determinations until these levels are normal, declining, stable, or until the child reaches 6 yr of age.
   c. Class II children require Pb/EP determinations monthly in the summer and every 2 mo in other seasons. Testing intervals may be increased up to 6 mo depending on the Pb/EP levels and the child's age.
   d. Class Ib patients should receive monthly Pb/EP determinations until their Pb status is clear; determinations can be adjusted thereafter.
   e. Class Ia children require care for the condition causing their elevated EP levels.

REFERENCES

Anemia
1. Dallman PR, Simes MA: Percentile curves for hemoglobin and red cell volume in infancy and childhood. *J Pediatr* 1979; 94:26-31.
2. Differential diagnosis of hypochromic microcytic anemia.- *Pediatric Oncology/Hematology Newsletter.* Vol.2 , Spring, 1979. Sidney Farber Cancer Institute, Boston.
3. Oski FA. Anemia in children. *Hosp Pract* 1976; 11:63-72.
4. Oski FA. Iron deficiency - facts and fallacies. *Ped Clin N Am* 1985; 32:493-497.
5. Oski FA: The non-hematologic manifestations of iron deficiency. *AJDC* 1979; 133:315-322.
6. Stockman JA, III: Office hematology: How valid are the results? *Contemp Pediatr* 1986; 21.

Hemophilia
1. Aledort LM: Current concepts in the diagnosis and management of hemophilia. *Hosp Pract* 1982; 17:77.
2. Karayalcin G: Current concepts in the management of hemophilia. *Pediatr Ann* 1985; 14:640.

Lead Poisoning
1. Mahaffery KR, Gartside PS, Glueck CJ: Blood lead levels and dietary calcium intake in 1 to 11 year old children. The second national health & nutrition examination survey, 1976 to 1980. Pediatr 198; 78:257-62.
2. *Preventing Lead Poisoning in Young Children,* Center for-Disease Control; Atlanta, Ga. US Dept of Health and Human Services, 1985.

Sickle Cell Disease
1. Pearson HA: Sickle cell diseases: diagnosis and management in infancy and childhood. *Pediatr in Rev* 1987; 9:121-130.

10

IMMUNIZATIONS

A. Routine

Recommended Schedule for Active Immunization of Normal Infants and Children

2 mo	DPT* TOPV
4 mo	DPT TOPV
6 mo	DPT/(OPV) optional for areas where polio might be imported
1 yr	Tuberculin Test (may be given simultaneously with the MMR at 15 mo)
15 mo	Measles, Mumps, Rubella (MMR)
18 mo	DPT TOPV
18 mo	Haemophilus influenzae type B vaccine (conjugated)
4-6 yr	DPT TOPV
14-16 yr	Td-repeat every 10 yrs**

*DPT should be administered to preterm infants and infants with intrauterine growth retardation when they reach a chronological age of 2 mo, regardless of their size.

**Combined tetanus and diphtheria toxoids (adult type) for those over 6 yr of age. Tetanus toxoid at time of injury. For clean minor wounds, no booster is needed by a fully immunized child unless more than 10 yr have elapsed since last dose. For contaminated wounds, a booster dose should be given if over 5 yr have elapsed since last dose.

B. Typical School Requirements (child cannot attend school without meeting these). These vary from state to state. Check the requirements in your area.

1. Elementary School
   a. Children younger than 6 yr of age.
      DPT - 4 doses (maximum of 5) with the last dose between ages 4-6 yr.
      OPV - 3 doses with the last dose between ages 4-6 yr.
      Measles - 1 dose on or after 15 months or a measles titer of 1:4 or greater (a history of having had measles is not acceptable).
      Rubella - 1 dose of rubella vaccine or a rubella titer of 1:8 or greater (a history of having had rubella is not acceptable).
   b. Children 6 yrs and older
      The requirements are the same as above, except 3 doses of DPT and/or dT (maximum of 5) with the last dose after the 4th birthday is acceptable.

2. Secondary School (grades 7-12)
   Measles - 1 dose of vaccine on or after 15 months or a measles titer of 1:4 or greater.
   N.B.—It is now recommended that measles vaccine be repeated on entry to kindergarten or junior high school.

C. Catch Up Schedules

Recommended Immunization Schedules for Infants and Children Not Initially Immunized at Usual Recommended Times in Early Infancy

Timing	Preferred Schedule	"Alternatives			Comments
		#1	#2	#3	
First visit	DPT#1, OPV#1 Tuberculin test (PPD)	MMR, PPD	DPT#1, OPV#1, PPD	DPT#1, OPV#1, MMR, PPD	MMR should be given no earlier than 15 mo of age
1 mo after first visit	MMR	DPT#1 OPV#1	MMR, DPT#2	DPT#2	
2 mo after first visit	DPT#2, OPV#2	- OPV#2	DPT#3, OPV#2	DPT#2	-
3 mo after first visit	(DPT#3)	DPT#2, OPV#2	-	-	In preferred schedule, DPT#3 can be given if OPV#3 is not to be given until 10-16 mo.
4 mo after first visit	DPT#3 (OPV#3)	-	(OPV#3)	(OPV#3)	OPV#3 optional in areas with likely importation of polio (e.g., some southwestern states
5 mo after first visit		DPT#3 (OPV#3)	-	-	
10-16 mo after last	DPT#4, OPV#3, or OPV#4	DPT#4, OPV#3 or DPT#4	DPT#4, OPV#3 or OPV#4	DPT#4, OPV#3 or OPV#4	-
Preschool	DPT#5, OPV#4 or OPV#5	DPT#5, OPV#4 or OPV#5	DPT#5, OPV#4 or OPV#5	DPT#5, OPV#4 or OPV#5	Preschool dose not necessary if DPT#4 or #5 given after fourth birthday.
14-16 yr old	Td	Td	Td	Td	Repeat every 10 yr.

A lapse in the immunization schedule generally does not require reinstitution of the entire series. If any of the first 3 doses of DPT or the first two doses of OPV had been given and the child failed to report for the next scheduled immunization, subsequent doses can be given at any interval after the first doses.

D. Miscellaneous

1. Live virus vaccines should not be given to immun-odeficient or immunosuppressed individuals (or close contacts) or patients being treated with steroids, antimetabolites, or radiation. Bacterial and inactivated viral vaccines (i.e., influenza) may be given, but the response may be inadequate.

2. For asymptomatic infants who are HIV positive, it is safer to use inactivated polio vaccine (Salk) at 2, 4, 18 mo and 4-6 yr, in place of the Sabin live virus vaccine. MMR vaccine should be given to both asymptomatic and symptomatic HIV-positive children.

3. Pertussis vaccine is contraindicated in children with evidence of progressive neurologic disease or in those patients who developed (1) screaming spells lasting >3 hr, (2) temperature of 105°F or greater, (3) hypotonia or excessive somnolence, (4) convulsion(s), (5) severe alteration of consciousness, (6) generalized and/or local neurologic signs, or (7) systemic allergic reaction following pertussis vaccine. In such cases, "splitting" of the vaccine dose is not indicated. A family history of convulsions is not a contraindication to pertussis vaccine.

4. It is now recommended to reimmunize children who received measles vaccine prior to 15 months.

5. It is safe to give rubella vaccine to the child of a pregnant woman, even if there is no maternal his-

tory of rubella or rubella immunization.

E. Non-routine Immunizations

1. Pneumococcal vaccine (pneumovax)
   a. Recommended for use in children over age 2 yr at high risk to develop severe pneumococcal infections. These include children with functional and anatomic asplenia (i.e., SS disease) and nephrotic syndrome.
   b. Given as single dose (0.5 cc). Boosters not recommended.
2. Influenza Vaccine
   a. Recommended for children over 6 mo of age with underlying heart, pulmonary, or other serious chronic disease for whom influenza may be a disaster.
   b. "Split-Product" (Subvirion) vaccine (less antigenic) is indicated for children under 13 yr.
   c. Initial series consists of 2 doses, 4 wk apart, followed by yearly booster.
   d. Should not be given to individuals with hypersensitivity to eggs.
3. Hepatitis B Vaccine
   a. Indicated in: institutionalized retarded children, users of illicit injectable drugs, male homosexuals, frequent recipients of blood/blood products (hemophiliacs), and sexual contacts of hepatitis B carriers.
   b. Use in children with household contact to hepatitis B carrier is controversial. Probably indicated if contact is chronic carrier (Hbs Ag-positive for over 6 mo), and child is in close contact (i.e., <5 yr of age).
   c. Babies born of HB_5Ag-positive mothers should receive 0.5 cc hepatitis B immune globulin (HBIG) within 12 hours of birth, in addition to immunization with HB vaccine (10 micrograms) within 7 days and repeated at 1 and 6 mo. The

initial dose can be given at the same time as the HBIG, but at a different site.)
4. Passive Immunization
   a. Immune Serum Globulin (ISG)
      1) For close personal exposure to a hepatitis A case, including day care exposure. Not indicated for usual casual school exposure.
      2) Dose is 0.02 cc/kg IM.
   b. Hepatitis B Immune Globulin (HBIG)
      1) After exposure to contaminated needles (0.06 cc/kg IM - repeat in 4 wk).
      2) For newborn infants born to Hepatitis B cases or chronic carriers 0.5 cc in the delivery room (may be effective even if delayed for up to 7 days).
   c. Varicella-Zoster Immune Globulin (VZIG)
      1) Indicated for immunocompromised susceptibles (including leukemia and lymphoma) closely exposed to varicella or zoster, including newborn infants whose mothers develop varicella rash 5 days or less prior to delivery or within 48 hr after delivery. Should be given within 72 hr of exposure.
      2) Dose is 1.25 cc/10 kg.

REFERENCES

1. CDC. Immunization of children infected with human-t-lymphotrophic virus type III/lymphadenopathy-associated virus. *MMWR* 1986; 35:595.
2. *1988 Redbook, Report of the Committee on Infectious Diseases*, 21st edition, American Academy of Pediatrics, Evanston, Illinois.

INGESTIONS

A. Telephone Triage

1. Many cases of ingestion will come to your attention by telephone call. Note time of call. Most parents will be frantic. You should remain calm.
2. Take a brief history. What was ingested? How much? (How many pills or how much liquid is missing?) When? Any vomiting? What is patient's present status?
3. Assess urgency. Should parents come to ER asap or should emergency vehicle be dispatched? If in doubt as to disposition, keep caller on hold and call local poison control center. Be sure to have parents bring ingested material with them plus the container.
4. Obtain name of caller, phone number, and address.
5. Advise emesis if the substance is not a caustic or hydrocarbon, and if the patient is not obtunded, comatose, or seizing.
   a. If emesis is indicated and parent has syrup of ipecac at home:
   The recommended dose is:

7-9 mo	-	5 cc
9-12 mo	-	10 cc
1-12 yr	-	15 cc
> 12 yr	-	30 cc

      b. Dose should be followed by 4-8 ounces of clear tepid fluids. Ipecac also works best if the patient is kept active.

      c. If there is no emesis in 15-20 minutes and the child is over 1 yr, repeat the dose x 1 (no more than once).

      N.B. Ipecac may not be effective after ingestion of anti-emetic substance.

  6. Instruct the parents to bring the child to the ER if any potentially dangerous substance has been ingested, or if the child is less than 6 mo of age.

B. Emergency Room Management

  1. Brief history (as above). If the nature of the ingestion is unknown, ask what medicines or other toxic substances (household products, kerosene, etc.) are in the house.

  2. Exam: note vital signs (T, P, R, BP), mental status, perfusion, respiratory status, pupils, unusual odors, any spills on clothes. (See *Harriet Lane Handbook* 11th ed., 1987).

  3. Lab:

      a. Urine (25-50 cc) is essential for toxicology screen; urine ferric chloride if appropriate.

      b. Blood (5-10 cc) for quantitation of substances picked up on urine screen and for detection of volatiles (alcohol, methanol, acetone).

      c. Talk to the lab - be sure its testing is set up to detect the specific agent you have in mind.

      d. Testing gastric aspirate does <u>not</u> identify what is in the child's blood, therefore, hold, pending results of urine screen.

      e. Consider Pb/FEP levels on all children <5 yr with ingestion.

  4. Induce emesis, if indicated (see dosage above).

      a. If there is no emesis in 15-20 minutes, repeat the dose x1.

      b. Ipecac generally works better than lavage; it can remove 25-30% of ingested toxin.

    c. Ipecac should <u>not</u> be given concurrently with charcoal, which will bind ipecac.

    d. Drowsiness will occur in 20% of patients. Rarely, there may be protracted vomiting.

    e. Ipecac should be avoided in patients with severe cardiac disease.

    f. Do not give ipecac if the patient is drowsy, obtunded, or at risk of rapid deterioration (i.e., tricyclic ingestion).

5. Gastric lavage

    a. If there is no response to ipecac or an emetic is contraindicated, insert a large-bore orogastric or nasogastric tube. Cutting large holes in the tube will facilitate removel of tablet or capsule fragments.

    b. Lavage with copious amounts (15 cc/kg/cycle) of warm normal saline until the return is clear. May need 5-10 liters.

    c. Patient should be in the Trendelenburg and left lateral decubitus position.

    d. If activated charcoal is to be given, administer <u>prior</u> to lavage and afterwards. Obtain gastric sample for analysis first.

    e. Contraindications to lavage include:

        1) ingestion of caustics and hydrocarbons.

        2) coma, seizures, or other impairment of airway protective mechanisms. If lavage is mandatory in such cases, it can be carried out after intubation with a cuffed endotracheal tube.

6. Activated Charcoal

This is probably the most effective GI decontamination procedure for most acute ingestions. No significant side effects. It is effective in preventing absorption of a toxin and also in promoting its excretion from the body ("GI dialysis"). It is especially effective if there is a delay between time of ingestion and gastric emptying.

a. Very effective for phenobarbital, theophylline, tricyclics, dextropropoxyphene, Digoxin, and salicylates.

b. <u>Not</u> effective for iron, strong acids and alkalis, and simple alcohols.

c. Charcoal should also be withheld following acetaminophen ingestion if oral N-acetylcysteine is to be used as an antidote, unless there is a mixed ingestion that is equally toxic. Also, do not use in cases where bicarbonate lavage is planned (i.e., iron poisoning).

d. Charcoal is usually given as a slurry in water; fruit juice may be added without loss of efficacy. Best placed in opaque container (cardboard orange juice container) to hide ugly appearance. If refused, it can be given via nasogastric or orogastric tube.

e. Usual dose is 1 gm/kg (minimum 30 gm). If the amount of toxin ingested is known, give 10x as much charcoal.

f. In cases that involve enterohepatic circulation (i.e., theophylline overdose), repeated doses may provide effective GI dialysis.

g. A cathartic such as sorbitol, magnesium sulfate, or magnesium citrate should be given along with or following charcoal to prevent constipation. There are preparations available that combine charcoal and sorbitol.

h. Suggested Protocol
   1) Administer charcoal/cathartic after emesis.
   2) Repeat half the initial dose (without cathartic) q 4 h until blood level is non-toxic, or there is absence of clinical toxicity.
   3) Administer cathartic q 12 h if patient has not had a stool.

7. Cathartics
   a. Efficacy questioned but frequently used.
   b. Dose: Magnesium citrate 3 - 4 ml/kg to maximum of 8 ounces.

Magnesium sulfate - 250 mg/kg of 10%
solution to 15-20 gm maximum.
Sorbitol - premixed with charcoal.
Magnesium-containing cathartic should
be avoided in patients with potential
nephrotoxicity.

c. Repeat q 4-6 h until there is passage of liquid
stool or any administered charcoal.

d. Cathartics should not be given following ingestion of caustics, in case of GI irritation that
occurs with iron poisoning, or if bowel sounds
are absent.

C. Specific Ingestions

There are too many toxins ingested by children to list
in this section. Since management changes from year
to year, listing specific information is pointless. The
best resource is your local poison control center,
which can provide up-to-date information regarding
management. Outlined below are some of the more
common ingestions.

1. Acetaminophen

a. Rapid intestinal absorption. Peak plasma level
in 70-120 minutes. May be earlier (30 minutes)
with liquid preparations in children.

b. Assessment of Risk:

1) Amount ingested 70-140 mg/kg: no treatment; hepatotoxicity is rare; give ipecac at
home.

2) Toxic dose in children: >140 mg/kg; ipecac at
home and send to ER.

c. Single plasma level is not reliable before 4 hr. If
the 4 h level is >300 mcg/cc, 90% chance of
severe toxicity. If the level is <150 mcg/cc, toxicity is unlikely, (Fig 11-1).

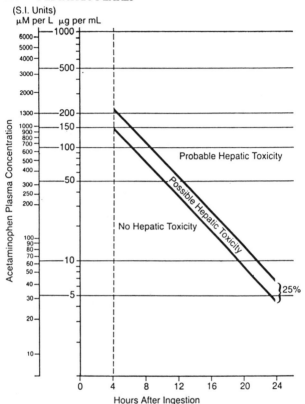

FIG 11 – 1. Rumack-Matthew nomogram for acetaminophen poisoning. Semi-logarithmic plot of plasma acetaminophen levels versus time. *Cautions for the use of this chart:* (1) the time coordinates refer to time after *ingestion.* (2) Serum levels drawn before 4 hr may not represent peak levels. (3) The graph should be used only in relation to a single acute ingestion. (4) The lower solid line 25% below the standard nomogram is included to allow for possible errors in acetaminophen plasma assays and estimated time from ingestion of an overdose. (From Rumack BH: POISINDEX: A COMPUTERIZED POISON INFORMATION SYSTEM. Ed 47. Micromedex, Inc., Denver, CO, 1986. Used by permission.

d. Treatment consists of emesis or gastric lavage followed by oral administration of N-acetylcysteine (effective within 14-16 hr of ingestion).
   1) Activated charcoal <u>should not</u> be administered.
   2) The oral protocol takes 72 hr. It may be associated with vomiting.
   3) The IV route of administration of N-acetylcysteine is faster and preferable, but not available for use in U.S. N-acetylcysteine can be made more palatable by putting it in juice, on ice, in a covered glass with a straw, (Fig 11-2).

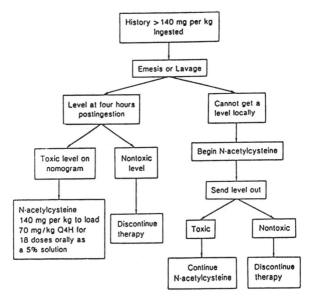

FIG 11 – 2. — Acetaminophen poisioning: treatment protocol. (From Peterson RG, Rumack BH: *Topics Emerg Med* 1979; Used by permission.)

  e. AST, ALT, bilirubin, and prothrombin time should be followed daily in all patients with levels in the toxic range.

  f. Prognosis

  1) Significant toxicity is rare in children <6 yr.

  2) Adolescents have a higher incidence of toxic plasma levels following ingestion, and one-third of those with toxic levels are likely to develop SGOT >1000 iu/L.

  3) Even with serious hepatotoxicity, mortality rate is <0.5%. Patients who recover have no sequelae.

2. Hydrocarbons

  a. These include gasoline, kerosene, lamp oil, lighter fluid, turpentine, paint thinner and remover, furniture polish, paraffin wax, and lubricating oil.

  b. Because of bad taste, large volumes are rarely ingested - usually < 1 ounce.

  c. Pulmonary injury results from aspiration not gastrointestinal absorption. Aspiration can occur in the absence of vomiting. Not indicated to evacuate gastric contents unless the material is contaminated by heavy metals, pesticides, or other toxins. Activated charcoal and cathartics are <u>not</u> indicated.

  d. Signs and symptoms include: coughing, choking, hemoptysis, tachypnea, dyspnea, cyanosis, rales, rhonchi, and wheezes. Somnolence is the chief neurologic manifestation (probably related to hypoxia and acidosis). High fever is common and does not correlate with infection. Respiratory symptoms almost always begin within 6 hr of ingestion.

  e. All patients should be observed for at least 6 hr. CXR is indicated only for those patients who are symptomatic; 90% of positive x-rays become so within 4 hours; they may show evidence of aspiration pneumonia, patchy densities, consolidation, hyperinflation, atelectasis, or pneumatoceles.

f. All symptomatic patients should be admitted. May be rapid deterioration over 24-48 hr.

g. Treatment is supportive. Steroids are not effective and prophylactic antibiotics are not indicated. Even in patients with fever and leukocytosis, bacterial pneumonia is unusual.

h. Course usually lasts 3-8 days. May be fever up to 8-10 days. CXR may show pneumatoceles 2-3 wk post-ingestion.

3. Iron

   a. Toxic dose of elemental iron is in the range of 20-50 mg/kg. A serum iron level drawn within 4 hr of ingestion is the best predictor of potential toxicity.

     1) >300 mcg/dl: intoxication likely.

     2) >500 mcg/dl: lethal range.

   b. Diagnosis

     If the clinical picture is consistent with iron poisoning, ingestion can be confirmed by:

     1) History - always assume that the maximum number of tablets missing was ingested.

     2) Abdominal x-ray for iron tablets and fragments.

     3) Combine 2 cc of gastric fluid and 2 drops of 30% H_2O_2 with 0.5 cc of deferoxamine solution (500 mg ampule) in 4 cc distilled water. The color will vary from light orange to dark red with increasing amounts of iron.

     4) Give one IM dose of deferoxamine (desferal) (50 mg/kg up to 1 gram). Pink (vin rose) color to urine indicates that the serum iron level exceeds the total iron-binding capacity (TIBC) and is high enough to produce toxicity.

   c. Clinical Features

     There are 4 phases of iron poisoning:

     1) 1/2-1 hr post-ingestion-hemorrhagic gastroenteritis (vomiting and bloody diarrhea), fever, metabolic acidosis, coagulation defects, shock, coma.

N.B. If signs and symptoms of toxicity do not appear within 4-6 hr, the process is unlikely to progress.

    2) 6-24 hr - period of relative improvement (may be the calm before the storm!).

    3) 24-48 hr - delayed profound shock, acidosis, pulmonary edema, hepatic failure, bleeding diathesis, renal shutdown, coma.

    4) 1-2 mo - gastric scarring; pyloric obstruction.

  d. Management

    1) Induce emesis with syprup of ipecac (if patient is alert).

    2) Gastric lavage with half-normal saline, 1% sodium bicarbonate or deferoxamine (2 gm) added to 1.5% bicarbonate solution; 100-150 cc of 1% sodium bicarbonate should be left in the stomach. Phosphate lavage, activated charcoal, and po deferoxamine <u>are not indicated.</u> An abdominal x-ray should be obtained post-lavage to check for retained fragments and tablets in stomach.

    3) Supportive care

      a) Correction of fluid and electrolyte abnormalities and acidosis

      b) Maintenance of intravascular volume - blood, colloid, and pressors

      c) Correction of clotting abnormalities

    4) Support of ventilation.

    5) Follow cbc, LFTs, clotting studies, electrolytes, ABGs, renal function.

    6) Chelation therapy with IV or IM deferoxamine. Indications include:

      a) Ingested dose of iron >25 mg/kg.

      b) Clinical evidence of severe toxicity.

      c) Serum iron exceeds TIBC (positive deferoxamine provocation test).

      d) Serum iron exceeds 300 mcg/dl 2-4 hr post-ingestion.

N.B. WBC >15000 and blood glucose >150 mg/dl

correlate with serum iron >300 mcg/dl and are suggestive of severe toxicity.

Chelation Protocol:

IM - 40 mg/kg (up to 1 gram) q 4-6 hr up to a maximum of 6 grams in 24 hr.

IV - 15 mg/kg/h by slow infusion in a solution of 100-200 cc D5W (This is the preferred route if patient is hypotensive). Dose may be repeated q 6 h depending on color of urine and patient's clinical status.

Chelation therapy is continued until disappearance of vin rose color from urine or serum iron level is less than TIBC.

7) If serum iron level >1000 mcg/cc or patient shows evidence of severe toxicity or renal shutdown, exchange transfusion or hemodialysis may be indicated.

4. Salicylate
  a. Clinical Picture
    1) Nausea, vomiting, fever, hyperpnea, tinnitus, coma, convulsions, hypoglycemia, oliguria, bleeding diathesis.
    2) Respiratory alkalosis (early) - metabolic acidosis (late).
    3) May be confused with DKA, Reye's syndrome, encephalitis, and other ingestions.
    4) Positive ferric chloride test (burgundy color change after 5-10 drops of 10% ferric chloride are added to urine that has been boiled for 1-2 minutes) and positive phenistix test.
  b. Estimation of toxicity
    1) Dose Ingested (mg/kg) Expected Toxicity

Dose Ingested (mg/kg)	Expected Toxicity
< 150	none
150-300	mild-moderate
300-500	serious
>500	potentially lethal

    2) The Done nomogram (Fig 11-3), based on the serum salicylate level 6 or more hr post-ingestion, gives a useful estimate of potential severity.

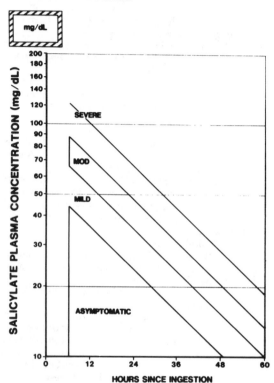

FIG 11 – 3. — Nomogram relating serum salicylate concentration and expected severity of intoxication at varying intervals following the ingestion of a single dose of salicylate. (From Done AK. *Pediatrics* 26:800-807, 1960. Used by permission.)

3) In acute overdose, peak serum level:

<35 mg/dl - no symptoms
35-70 mg/dl - mild-moderate symptoms
70-100 mg/dl - severe symptoms
>100 mg/dl - potentially fatal

    c. Management

        1) Hospitalization indicated if patient is symptomatic, or if peak serum level exceeds 50 mg/dl.

        2) Removal of gastric contents by syrup of ipecac (if patient is alert) or by gastric lavage.

        3) Activated charcoal/cathartic.

        4) IV replacement of fluid/electrolyte deficits-- aim for urine output of 3-6 cc/kg/h. Start with 10-15 cc/kg/h for first two hours and then adjust.

        5) Alkalinize the urine - give sodium bicarbonate, 2-3 mEq/kg as a loading dose, followed by 2 mEq/kg q 2-4 h to maintain urine pH above 8. Add 35-40 mEq/L of potassium to IV fluids. Follow urine pH and volume, plasma pH, serum glucose, LFTs, electrolytes, and prothrombin time.

        6) Vitamin K for prolonged prothrombin time.

        7) Hemodialysis and hemoperfusion are rarely needed. Indications include: renal failure, unresponsive acidosis, intractable seizures, coma, or a serum salicylate level >100 mg/dl.

5. Theophylline

    a. Manifestations include: agitation, obtundation, seizures, sinus tachycardia, arrythmias, vomiting.

    b. Difference in <u>acute</u> vs. <u>chronic</u> overdose

        1) In <u>acute</u> overdose, serious toxicity is unlikely with serum theophylline level <100 mcg/cc.

        2) In <u>chronic</u> overdose, serious toxicity can occur at levels <40 mcg/cc.

    c. Treatment

        1) Vigorous GI decontamination: syrup of ipecac or gastric lavage followed by activated charcoal and a cathartic.

        2) Activated charcoal can bind drug within the GI tract, prevent enterohepatic reabsorption, and increase drug clearance from within the

vascular compartment.

3) Charcoal can be given as multiple intermittent oral doses or as a continuous nasogastric infusion (0.5 gm/kg/hr), interrupted for one dose of magnesium citrate, and continued until the serum level is in the non-toxic range.

4) Hemodialysis or hemoperfusion indicated if serum level >100 mcg/cc in acute overdose or if patient fails to respond to supportive care.

5) Seizures should be treated with IV diazepam.

6. Tricyclic Antidepressants (TCA)

   a. Manifestations are those of autonomic dysfunction: fever, dry mouth, tachycardia, flushing, dilated pupils, excitation along with confusion, arrythmias, hallucinations, hypotension, seizures, and coma. The triad of anticholinergic signs, acute alteration of mental status, and sinus tachycardia suggests tricyclic poisoning. Prolongation of the QRS complex (> 100 m sec) has been correlated with severe overdoses. However, this finding will miss a substantial portion of patients with CNS toxicity and will include many patients who never develop serious problems.

   b. Blood levels are not usually helpful in acute ingestions-treatment should be based on the clinical picture.

   c. Even if the patient is alert, do not give syrup of ipecac. Carry out gastric lavage. If the patient is not alert, lavage with a cuffed endotracheal tube in place. This should be followed by activated charcoal/cathartic regimen.

   d. All symptomatic patients should be admitted to an intensive care unit for supportive management and cardiac monitoring.

      1) Support blood pressure and cardiac output.

      2) Diazepam for seizures.

      3) Correction of acidosis and electrolyte disturbances.

      4) Management of arrhythmias.

    e. Physostigmine and dialysis - not usually indicated.

    f. A depressed level of consciousness (Glasgow-coma scale <8) is the best predictor of serious complications of TCA overdose. Significant complications almost always occur within 3 1/2 hr of ingestion. Patients who remain awake after observation in the ER are at low risk for serious complications.

D. Household Product Ingestion

Be suspicious of this type of ingestion if:

1. 1-5 yr old patient with a previous history of ingestion.
2. Nonfebrile illness; multisystem involvement without obvious explanation.
3. Unusual odor, stains on clothing, burns around mouth or on oral mucosa.
4. Unexplained hematemesis.

E. Munchausen by Proxy

1. "Accidental" ingestion may not be accidental. Some children may be abused (usually by the mother) by the administration of drugs. In many cases, the abuse continues while the patient is in the hospital. The abuser is often pleasant, cooperative, and appreciative.
2. Be suspicious if:
   a. Child is <1 or >5 yr
   b. More than one ingestion episode
   c. Bizarre clinical manifestations
   d. Risk factors for abuse are present

REFERENCES

1. Anas N, Namasonth V, Ginsburg CM: Criteria for hospitalizing children who have ingested products containing hydrocarbons. *JAMA* 1981; 246:840-843.

2. Arena JM: Hydrocarbon poisoning - current management. *Pediatr Annals* 1987; 16:879-883.

3. Banner W Jr, Tong TG: Iron poisoning. *Pediatr Clin N Am* 1986; 33:393-410.

4. Braden NJ, Jackson JE, Walson PD: Tricyclic antidepressant overdose. *Pediatr Clin N Am* 1986; 33:287-297.

5. Committee on Accident and Poison Prevention, American Academy of Pediatrics. *Handbook of Common Poisonings in Children,* 2nd edition, Aronow R, Ed., Evanston, Illinois, 1983.

6. Haddad LM: The emergency management of poisoning. *Pediatr Annals* 1987; 16:900-912.

7. Klein BL, Simon JE: Hydrocarbon poisoning. *Pediatr Clin N Am* 1986; 33:411-419.

8. Krenzelok EP, Dean BS: Syrup of ipecac in children less than one year of age. *Clinical Toxicology* 1985; 23:171-176.

9. Litovitz TL, et al: Ipecac administration in children younger than one year of age. *Pediatr* 1985; 76:761-764.

10. Meadow R: Munchausen by proxy. *Arch Dis Child* 1982; 57:92.

11. Riggs BS, Kulig K, Rumack BH: Current status of aspirin and acetaminophen intoxication. *Pediatr Annals* 1987; 16:886-898.

12. Rodgers GC Jr, Matyunas NJ: Gastrointestinal decontamination for acute poisoning. *Pediatr Clin N Am* 1986; 33:261-285.

13. Rumack BH: Acetaminophen overdose in children. *Pediatr Clin N Am* 1986; 33:691-701.

14. Snodgrass WR: Salicylate toxicity. *Pediatr Clin N Am* 1986; 33:381-392.

12

NEONATAL PROBLEMS

A. Blocked Nasolacrimal (tear) duct

1. Due to obstruction at the distal end of the duct, usually unilateral.
2. Usually appears between 2nd and 3rd wk of life.
   a. Constant tearing.
   b. Accumulation of dried mucoid material at inner canthus.
   c. Secondary conjunctivitis due to reflux of purulent material.
3. Treatment - Daily massage of sac at root of nose; the duct usually opens spontaneously by 6-9 mo. If obstruction persists past 9 mo, refer to ophthalmologist for probing (under general anesthesia) of the duct.
   N.B. Diff Dx of unilateral tearing includes congenital glaucoma.

B. Breast Engorgement

Breast engorgement 2° to transfer of maternal hormones is physiologic in newborn infants. It is usually bilateral and may be associated with breast secretions. Peak enlargement (1-3 cm) may not be reached until 4-6 wk and may persist for several mo. No Rx is indicated.

C. Breast Infection

1. Most frequent during 2nd-3rd wk. Presents as <u>unilateral</u> firm swelling with tenderness and warmth. Systemic manifestations, except for low-grade fever, are rare.
2. May be helpful to aspirate material for gram stain and culture - usually due to <u>S. aureus.</u>
3. Admit for IV antistaphylococcal therapy. I + D may be needed.

D. Constipation

1. Defined by character of stools (hard and dry) and not frequency. Number of stools can be very variable ranging from 8-10/d to 1 every 3-4 days, even in nursing infants.
2. Causes include inadequate milk intake and the switch from breast to bottle. Consider hypothyroidism and Hirschsprung's disease. Rectal exam indicated. Look for anal fissure, tight anal sphincter, and lack of stool in rectum (Hirschsprung's).
   N.B. Almost all cases of Hirschsprung's are symptomatic by 4 wk of age.
3. If specific etiologies are ruled out, Rx by adding 1 tsp sugar to formula, adding 4-6 oz of glucose water/day, or by occasionally using glycerine suppositories.

E. Omphalitis

1. During the first wk, faint erythema of the rim of the umbilical stump is common and of no consequence.
2. Omphalitis is defined by:
   a. Foul-smelling discharge,
   b. Periumbilical erythema and induration,
   c. Purulent or sero-sanguinous drainage.
3. Treatment
   a. With purulent discharge or periumbilical involvement - use oral or parenteral antibiotics based on C + S.

    b. Without periumbilical spread - use topical antibiotic.

N.B.   a. With serous umbilical secretion, you need to R/O vitelline duct or urachal remnant.

        b. Wet malodorous stump with minimal inflammation can be seen with group A ß-hemolytic strep infection.

F. Rashes

1. Acropustulosis

   Recurrent crops of pruritic vesiculopustules on the hands and feet, lasting 7-10 days, and recurring every few wk to mo over the first 2 to 3 yr. Gram stain reveals numerous polys and occasional eosinophils. The etiology is unknown and there is no specific therapy. Antihistamines can be used for relief of pruritus.

2. Bullous Disease

   Several varieties of epidermolysis bullosa have onset in the neonatal period with bullae involving the skin and mucous membranes. These often occur at sites of trauma. Any bullous lesions (blistering) in the neonatal period require immediate dermatologic consultation.

3. Erythema Toxicum

   Evanescent papules, vesicles, and pustules on an erythematous base occurring on the face, forehead, chest, trunk, and extremities (not palms and soles) of a high percentage of full-term newborns. They usually have onset between 24-72 hr but may be seen at birth. Gram stain of contents reveals sheets of eosinophils. They resolve over 3 to 5 days without therapy.

4. Miliaria (Prickly heat)

   Pruritic, erythematous 1 to 2 mm papulovesicular lesions with predilection for clothed and intertriginous areas of the body. Gram stain of the contents is negative. They may occur during the first few wk of life. Treatment consists of less heat, less clothing, and cool soaks.

5. Neonatal Lupus Syndrome

Lesions consist of erythematous, oval-shaped (discoid), slightly atrophic macules with peripheral scaling. May appear from birth up to 12 wk. Primarily localized to the head (periorbital areas) and neck. May be associated with anemia, leukopenia, thrombocytopenia. Congenital A-V block occurs in 15% of cases. Serum is positive for antibodies to Ro antigen. Most cases are transient with resolution of skin lesions by 6 mo, <u>but</u> disease may progress to subacute or acute SLE.

6. Pustular Melanosis

Presents at or shortly after birth as brownish 3 to 4 mm vesicles and pustules on the neck, face, palms, and soles. Within a few days the pustules shed, leaving pigmented macules with scaling. Gram stain reveals sheets of polys. Lesions tend to recur in crops, but gradually resolve by 3 to 4 mo without scarring. Condition is seen mainly in blacks. The etiology is unknown and there is no treatment.

7. Pustulosis (Neonatal impetigo)

a. Small vesicles to larger bullae-rupture easily leaving a red, moist, denuded base that crusts over. They occur in periumbilical and diaper areas with onset at 7-10 days of age. Usually due to <u>S. aureus</u>.

b. Gram stain and culture fluid. Start an oral antistaphylococcal agent (Dicloxacillin, Cephalexin). Lesions will usually clear in 5-7 days. Most patients can be treated at home. It is rarely associated with systemic manifestations.

N.B. It is important to report all cases to nursery of origin - may be harbinger of staph outbreak in nursery.

G. Thrush

1. Oral candidiasis has peak incidence during 2nd wk of life.
2. Cheesy white plaques on an erythematous base over gingiva, tongue, palate, and buccal mucosa - cannot be easily removed.
3. Often associated with candidal diaper rash.
4. Rx: Nystatin suspension 100,000-200,000 units po-qid x 7-10 days.

   N.B. In breast-fed infant, may help to have mother apply mycostatin cream to areola/nipple area.

   If thrush is recurrent or refractory to treatment, consider workup for endocrinopathy or immuno-deficiency (? AIDS).

H. Umbilical Granuloma

1. Cord usually separates by 8-10 days (2-3 days later after C-section) and heals within 3-5 days. Delayed separation and/or mild infection may result in moist granulating area at base of cord with slight mucoid discharge. Treat with alcohol swabs several times a day.
2. Occasionally may be persistence of reddish-pink, soft, granular-meaty tissue (granuloma) protruding from base of umbilicus. Treatment consists of single application of silver nitrate cautery - be careful to swab only over area of granuloma.
3. With persistent drainage of fluid or (?) stool from umbilicus, consider patent omphalomesenteric duct or urachus.

   N.B. Marked delay in cord separation may be clue to granulocyte dysfunction.

I. Umbilical Hernia

1. Central fascial defect due to imperfect closure of umbilical ring. May be pinpoint size to >5 cm. Easily reduced. Incarceration is possible but rare. Common

in blacks and premature infants. Also associated with hypotonia, i.e., Down's syndrome, hypothyroidism.

2. Most hernias close spontaneously by 2-3 yr. Surgery not indicated unless >5 cm or still large past 5 yr. Pressure or adhesive dressings with coins and metallic or plastic objects are popular but useless (may lead to contact dermatitis).

   N.B. If there is progressive enlargement of the skin over the umbilicus until a downward-pointing proboscis is formed, surgical repair will probably be needed.

J. Vaginal Discharge/Bleeding

1. During the first wk of life, a thick, milky-white vaginal discharge and vaginal bleeding (due to estrogen withdrawal) are not uncommon. Reassurance only is indicated.

2. Older infants may develop labial adhesions secondary to mild irritation. See p. 116.

REFERENCES

Neonatal Problems
1. Findlay RF, Odom RB: Infantile acropustulosis. *Am J Dis Child* 1983; 137:455.
2. Watson R: Neonatal lupus syndrome. *Pediatr Annals* 1986; 15:605-620.

13

NEUROLOGY

A. Altered Mental Status

1. Altered mental status includes any change in sensorium or behavior. In extreme cases it includes stupor/coma and hyperirritability. In milder cases, it may be manifested by confusion, sleepiness, aggressive behavior, and decreased school or social performance.
2. Important historical information includes:
   a. A complete description of the alteration of sensorium (onset, acute or gradual, duration, waxing and waning vs progressive).
   b. Previous mental state.
   c. Possible precipitating events, psychological stress, medication, or illicit drug use.
   d. Signs of illness, especially fever.
   e. Chronic medical condition.
   f. History of trauma, depression, change in school or social performance.
   g. Presence of headaches, visual disturbances.
3. The PE must be thorough. Special emphasis should be placed on the neurologic exam, fundoscopic assessment, nuchal rigidity, and skin findings (herpetic lesions, bruises, etc). Note odor on breath.
4. Causes of altered mental status

      a. CNS infection (meningitis, encephalitis).
      b. CNS masses (usually gradual onset of symptoms).
      c. CNS hemorrhages (may be acute or gradual and may be preceded by headache) or infarcts.
      d. CNS trauma.
      e. Medication/drug overdose.
      f. Illicit drug use, including alcohol.
      g. Hypertensive encephalopathy.
      h. Hypoglycemia.
      i. Diabetic ketoacidosis.
      j. Reye's syndrome.
      k. Depression.
      l. Postictal state.

5. Laboratory tests are dictated by the history, PE, and the type of mental status change.
   a. For the comatose, stuporous, hyperirritable patient, serum electrolytes, cbc, serum glucose, and a toxicology screen should be obtained.
   b. If vital signs are stable and there are no localizing neurologic signs or evidence of increased intracranial pressure, an LP should be considered (CSF sent for glucose, protein, Gram stain, cell count, and culture/ELISA).
   c. In the unstable patient or with localized neurologic signs, a CT scan may need to precede the LP.
6. Treatment is tailored to the underlying cause of the altered mental status.

B. Headache

1. Headache is a very common presenting complaint, especially in the older pediatric age group and in febrile children.
2. Important historical information includes:
   a. The headache's location, day(s) and time(s) of occurrence, frequency, duration, precipitating factors, ameliorating factors and associated

symptoms (fever, neck pain, scotoma, photo-phobia, nausea, vomiting, etc).
  b. Does the patient have a chronic medical condition or take medications on a chronic basis?
  c. Is there a family history of headaches? If so, who has them and what are their headaches like?
  d. Does the patient have a history of head trauma, seizures, cranial surgery, allergies, decreased vision or hearing, or pain on chewing? Has his headache ever awakened him from sleep?
  e. Is the patient stressed? Have there been changes in his personality, school performance, or growth?
3. Physical exam should be complete. Place emphasis on the skull, eyes, ears, teeth, temporomandibular joints, sinuses, and the neurologic exam. Look for areas of tenderness, asymmetry, bruits.
4. No single laboratory test is mandatory for the patient who presents with a headache. Laboratory tests and x-ray studies should be dictated by the results of the history and physical examination.
5. Frontal headaches may be due to viral illnesses, especially when accompanied by fever; sinus infection; sinus edema (due to exposure to allergens or noxious environmental stimuli such as smoke); stress; or fatigue.
  a. Presence of pain upon palpation of the sinuses and a purulent nasal discharge suggest sinusitis; a radiograph may confirm the diagnosis.
  b. Presence of suborbital edema/cyanosis, enlarged bluish nasal turbinates, or watery ocular/nasal discharge suggest allergic disease.
6. Facial pain may be due to dental disease; middle ear disease; temporomandibular joint dysfunction, or maxillary sinusitis.
7. Pain in the temples or neck pain (tightness) may be due to stress (especially if the pain occurs during stressful situations) or depression.

8. Occipital headaches may be associated with intracranial disease (bleeds, tumors, abscesses, pseudotumor cerebri). This is especially true if the pain occurs upon arising in the morning, is relieved by vomiting, and is accompanied by visual field or acuity changes, or alterations in mental status, mood, motor function, or sensation.

9. Generalized (or poorly localized) headaches may be due to fatigue; stress; medications, such as sympathomimetics; illicit drugs, such as amphetamines; encephalitis (frequently associated with sensorium changes); meningitis (usually associated with positive Kernig and Brudzinski signs); severe anemia; hypertension; hyperventilation; hypoglycemia; hypoxia; hypercapnia; carbon monoxide poisoning; and trauma.

   a. A severe headache may herald a cerebral aneurysm; this is especially true if the patient is confused or unconscious.

10. Migraine headaches are "classically" paroxysmal, unilateral, and preceded by an aura or accompanied by nausea and vomiting. Not all patients present with classic symptoms. Younger children may present with abdominal pain and vomiting. A family history of migraine is helpful for diagnosis.

11. Treatment of uncomplicated headaches includes analgesics and rest.

    a. Headaches due to bacterial processes respond to antibiotic therapy of the underlying disease.

    b. Headaches due to allergen exposure respond to the elimination of the offending agent; antihistamines may be useful if other histamine-mediated symptoms are present.

    c. Headaches due to stress or depression respond to the elucidation and resolution of the psychic conflict.

    d. Headaches due to mass intracranial lesions or bleeds are treated surgically.

    e. Once a migraine headache is firmly established,

it cannot be treated; however, use of propranolol (80 mg po qd) for children $\geq$ 12 yr) can prevent episodes or abort a headache if taken early in its course. Other helpful modalities include biofeedback and counseling.

C. Head Trauma

1. Evaluation

   The main objective is to sort out patients who have treatable complications (e.g., intracranial bleeding, depressed fractures) from those who do not. This can be difficult.

   a. The history should include details on the type of trauma (fall, blow, etc.) described in detail, loss of consciousness, duration of loss, amnesia (especially retrograde), lethargy, vomiting, seizures, vision difficulties, and history of other medical problems (especially shunt). Many patients will have a period of sleepiness, headaches, and vomit a few times without sequelae. Think about the possibility of child abuse.

   b. The exam should be complete, including vital signs with BP (increased intracranial pressure causes ↓ pulse, ↑ BP, irregular respirations); look for direct signs of trauma - soft tissue swelling, hematoma, depression of skull, and lacerations. Pay particular attention to:

      1) Fundus - retinal hemorrhage; papilledema (usually a <u>late</u> sign of ↑ICP). Do not use mydriatics to dilate pupils.
      2) TMs - blood behind drum or CSF discharge.
      3) Ecchymosis - behind ear (Battle sign) or orbital (raccoon sign); basilar skull fracture.
      4) Nose - CSF rhinorrhea.
      5) Neck exam - make sure cervical spine isn't injured. If in doubt, stabilize head with sandbags or neck collar and obtain C-spine films.
      6) Skin - check for signs of abuse.

    7) Neurologic exam - emphasize level of consciousness and general mental state - serial observations mandatory.
- a) Eyes - unequal pupils signifies compression of 3rd nerve by herniating temporal lobe.
- b) Diplopia - 6th nerve (to lateral rectus) is particularly vulnerable to ↑ICP.
- c) Motor - use of arms and legs normal? Ataxic gait?
- d) Reflexes - symmetric? Toes go down?

  c. Level of consciousness probably most important observation.

  d. X-rays
- 1) Skull x-rays are expensive and overutilized. In general, fractures are poor predictors of intracranial injury. Patient management is rarely affected by radiologic findings.
  - a) Skull x-rays are probably indicated in the following situations: Age <1 yr, unconscious >5 minutes, gunshot wound or skull penetration, V-P shunt in place, palpable scalp depression, CSF discharge from ear or nose, blood in middle ear, Battle sign, raccoon sign, lethargy, coma or stupor, and focal neurologic signs. In many of these cases, however, a CT scan may be the preferable study.
- 2) Don't forget C-spine stabilization and x-ray if head injury is severe, as in auto accident. Cervical abrasions or upper spine tenderness suggest neck injury.

  e. Order CT scan if intracranial bleed is suspected, i.e., patients with persistent or progressing neurologic signs.

  f. EEG is not indicated in initial evaluation and/or uncomplicated cases.

2. Management
  a. Send patient home when level of consciousness and function are back to normal.

b. If exam and level of consciousness are normal, give parents instructions for home care. Level of alertness should be evaluated every few hours for the first 24 hr. Parents should note any fever or change in mental status over the next 2 wk and return if problems develop.

c. Usually hospitalize if:
   1) Any sign of deterioration.
   2) Clear-cut neurologic signs.
   3) Prolonged loss of consciousness.
   4) Level of function does not return promptly to normal (sometimes these patients may be sent home if parents are reliable, overall exam is reassuring, and neurology consult agrees).
   5) Fracture across area of middle meningeal artery or depressed skull fx.

d. Seizure in the first 24 hr after the injury is not an automatic admission, nor is a skull fracture.

e. If any questions, get neurology consult.

f. Give parents written instructions for follow-up at home.

D. Increased Intracranial Pressure

1. Signs and symptoms include headache, nausea, vomiting, spectrum of altered mental status, and papilledema.
   a. NOTE vital signs and any change suggestive of Cushing's response (decreased pulse, slow respirations, increased BP with widening pulse pressure).
   b. Patient may be delirious and thrashing about, or may be completely obtunded with severe ↑ ICP.

2. Etiologies include trauma, infections, metabolic (Reye's syndrome), tumor, hypoxic/ischemic damage, and shunt malfunction.

3. Priorities are establishing and maintaining appropriate ventilation and perfusion, and decreasing ICP.

a. Controlled intubation and hyperventilation. Hyperventilation is the most rapid means to decrease ICP. If patient is obtunded, intubation should not be difficult nor require premedication (e.g., muscle relaxants). If patient is thrashing about, Valium 0.1-0.2 mg/kg IV push, should be adequate to allow intubation, and it will not increase ICP.

NOTE: Do not use pavulon, as this paralysis will prevent assessing neurologic status during first critical hours. Succinylcholine may lead to fatal hyperkalemia. Valium is a safe "relaxant" to use in ER setting until patient can be transferred to an intensive care unit.

b. Hypertonic Agents. Mannitol 0.5-1.0 gm/kg/ IV over 20 minutes will help decrease cerebral edema and thereby decrease ICP. Useful in initial emergency management.

OR (not b&c together)

c. Diuretic. Furosemide 1 mg/kg/dose IV (maximum 6 mg/kg) has both diuretic effect and independent effect on decreasing ICP (one effect is decreased CSF production).

E. CNS Infections

1. CNS infections include bacterial meningitis, aseptic meningitis, encephalitis, and brain abscesses.
   a. Patients with these processes may present with nuchal rigidity, headache, behavior changes, seizures, sensorium changes, focal neurologic signs, or fever.
   b. Depending on the agent causing the infection, other signs may be present (rash, vomiting, diarrhea, pneumonia, etc).
2. Important historical information includes eliciting the duration and character of any of the signs listed in #1. In the confused or comatose patient, a history of drug ingestion must also be sought.

3. A complete PE is mandatory with special emphasis on the neck (? nuchal rigidity), skull (? trauma, ? tenderness, ? split sutures), skin (? rash, especially petechiae/purpura), and the neurologic exam (? focal findings, sensorium, orientation, cranial nerves, etc.) The fundi must be visualized (to R/O papilledema) before a spinal tap is performed.

4. Laboratory tests are important diagnostic tools.
   a. Spinal fluid is examined for cell count, protein, glucose (to be compared with a simultaneous serum glucose), and organisms (Gram stain).
   b. Countercurrent immunoelectrophoresis (CIE) and latex particle agglutination tests of CSF, blood, and urine may help to rapidly diagnose <u>H. influenzae, S. pneumoniae, N. meningitidis</u>, and <u>Group B Streptococcus</u> infections.
   c. Blood and urine cultures should also be obtained.
   d. Serum electrolytes, BUN, creatnine, and a cbc with diff and smear may also be helpful.
   e. If an ingestion is suspected, a toxicology screen is indicated.
   f. If there are focal findings (i.e. if one suspects a brain abscess), an LP is contraindicated (herniation possible). Instead, an emergent CT scan is indicated.

5. a. Etiologies include bacterial meningitis: <u>H. influenzae, S. pneumoniae, N. meningiditis,</u> Group B <u>Streptococcus, Listeria, S. aureus,</u> and <u>Pseudomonas</u> (the latter 3 in neonates).
   b. Aseptic meningitis: most commonly enterovirus.
   c. Encephalitis: S/P measles, varicella, mumps, influenza, Epstein-Barr infections, herpes.
   d. Abscesses: <u>S. aureus</u>, Group A <u>Streptococcus, H. influenzae</u>, anaerobes, gram-negative enteric bacteria, fungi.

6. Treatment
   a. Brain abscess: Surgery/aspiration via Burr holes; fluid restriction; nafcillin/methicillin (200 mg/kg/d ÷ q 4-6 h) and chloramphenicol 100 mg/kg/d ÷ 6 h); dexamethasone (0.1-0.2 mg/kg/dose IV q 4h, up to 1.5 mg/kg/d). If severely elevated ICP, incline head of bed to 30°; mannitol (0.25-2g/kg/dose over 20 minutes), intubation, paralysis, hyperventilation (to keep PCO2 23-25), ICP monitoring, pentobarbital coma; phenobarbital or Dilantin if seizures.
   b. Aseptic meningitis: May need to give ampicillin (200-300 mg/kg/d ÷ q 4 h) and chloramphenicol (100 mg/kg/d ÷q 6 h) for 3 days pending negative cultures if CSF cell count is confusing or contaminated with blood; fluid restriction (to avoid SIADH); IV fluids, analgesics/antipyretics; incline head of bed 30°; if herpes encephalitis, acyclovir/vidarabine; phenobarbital/Dilantin for seizures.
   c. Bacterial meningitis: Ampicillin (200-300 mg/kg/d ÷ q 4 h) and chloramphenicol (100 mg/kg/d ÷q 6 h); may also use cefotaxime (200 mg/kg/d ÷q 6 h) or ceftriaxone (150 mg/kg/d ÷q 12 h) instead of chloramphenicol. If <u>S. pneumoniae</u> or <u>N. meningitidis</u> is the organism, penicillin G (300,000 u/kg/d ÷q 4 h) is used; follow vital signs and neurologic status carefully; restrict fluid (npo x 24 h and then total fluids - oral and IV - to 60-75% maintenance) to prevent SIADH. Follow head circumferences; may need CT scan to R/O subdural if (1) focal neurologic signs, (2) focal seizures, and (3) increasing head circumference. Phenobarbital (loading dose 15-25 mg/kg no faster than 30 mg/min; maintenance dose 4-6 mg/kg/d divided q 12 h) or Dilantin (loading dose 15-20 mg/kg in normal saline no faster than 50 mg/min, maintenance dose 4-7 mg/kg/d divided qd or q 12 h) for seizures.

F. **Seizures, Febrile Seizures, and Status Epilepticus**

1. Status epilepticus is a seizure that lasts 20 or more minutes or in which there is incomplete recovery between recurrent seizures. Immediate management includes the following.
   a. Stabilize the patient.
   b. Maintain airway and maximize ventilation (insert oral airway or intubate).
   c. Prevent aspiration (clear secretions with suctioning and insert NG tube to aspirate stomach).
   d. Restrain to avoid injury.
   e. Give O_2 (if indicated).
   f. Establish good IV access.
   g. If febrile, tepid sponging and rectal antipyretics may be helpful.

2. Important historical information to obtain when presented with a child with seizures.
   a. Assess if a real seizure occurred. (Need to assess if choking spell or breath-holding spell was more likely than a seizure).
   b. Prior seizures? Medications? Fever? Circumstances? Precipitating event? Hx. of drug abuse/ingestions? Trauma? Remember occult trauma (i.e., abuse).
   c. Main causes of seizures:

1) infants:	infection, febrile seizures, dehydration, electrolyte imbalance, birth injury, CNS malformations.
2) children:	head trauma, noncompliance or change of medication, intercurrent infection in known seizure patient, toxin ingestion (don't forget lead), tumor, febrile seizure.

3. Initial Evaluation
    a. Vital signs (T, P, R, BP).
    b. Any seizure activity? (Lateralization, eye deviation, focal vs. generalized).
    c. Exam: (quick and pertinent)
       Assess neurologic status (pupils, response, s/sx of increased ICP, fontanelle); cardiovascular (BP, perfusion); respiratory (cyanosis, irregular breathing, ineffective ventilation).
       NOTE breath odor, rash, signs of trauma, liver size, s/sx of infection (sepsis, meningitis).
       <u>Keep reassessing</u> - status may quickly change!
    d. Initial lab
       1) Dextrostix or chemstrip.
       2) Electrolytes, Ca, Glucose, BUN, cbc, anticonvulsant levels (if applicable).
       3) Toxicology screen on blood and urine (+vomitus if indicated).
       4) Sepsis workup including LP might be indicated.
       5) Consider need for LFTs; Mg; Pb; NH4+.
       6) CT scan might be indicated.
4. Treatment
    a. IV route preferred for all medications in status. If any possibility of hypoglycemia (√ dextrostix), IV bolus D25W 2-3 cc/kg, followed by continuous glucose infusion.
    b. Diazepam (Valium) 0.3 mg/kg to 0.5 mg/kg at rate of 1 mg/min by slow direct IV injection; may repeat q 15 min to total of 2 doses; avoid dose >5 mg in infants or >10 mg in older children.
       1) Advantage - rapidly effective.
       2) Disadvantages - respiratory depression. Drug quickly redistributed throughout the body and seizures may recur as this takes place. May cause cardiovascular and respiratory depression if the patient has been on barbiturate.

  3) Don't forget to place patient on longer-acting anticonvulsant. Use Dilantin or phenobarbital in most cases. Load as in c. or d. below, then place on maintenance dose.
 c. Phenytoin (Dilantin) 15-20 mg/kg in normal saline slowly at 1 to 3 mg/kg/ minute.
  1) Best to monitor ECG for arrhythmias when giving IV.
  2) Advantages - doesn't cloud consciousness (good for head trauma victims to help monitor mental status).
  3) Longer half-life than Valium.
  4) Disadvantages - seizures don't respond as quickly as with Valium.
 d. Phenobarbital 15-25 mg/kg IV, no faster than 30 mg/min. If seizures continue for 20-30 more minutes, give repeat dose of 10 mg/kg.
  Disadvantage - slow onset; takes up to 15 minutes to cross blood-brain barrier.
5. Febrile seizure: 2-5% of all children will develop febrile seizure.
 a. Onset: Most occur between 6 mo and 3 yr of age - up to 6 yr.
 b. Duration: 50% <5 minutes. 75% <20 minutes. Type: Most are clonic, generalized; 15% are focal.
 c. Most occur with temperature >39°C (102.2°F) and at onset of fever. Seizure that occurs after a fever has been present for more than 24 hr is more likely to be associated with significant infection.
 d. Treatment
  1) Diazepam and/or phenobarbital for acute control of status (dosages as given above).
  2) Reduce fever with tepid baths, rectal acetaminophen.
  3) Evaluate and treat underlying infection (see LP below).

    e. Continuous prophylactic anticonvulsant therapy following first febrile seizure is not generally recommmended. There is no evidence of mental or neurologic impairment due to febrile seizures.

    f. Consider prophylaxis if patient has high-risk factors for subsequent nonfebrile seizure:
      1) Seizure >15 minutes duration.
      2) Febrile seizure with focal component or associated with transient or persistent neurologic abnormalities.
      3) Presence of abnormal neurologic exam.
      4) Family hx of non-febrile seizures.

    g. There is no evidence that prophylaxis reduces the risk of subsequent non-febrile seizures.

    h. Do LP if:
      1) Any suspicion of meningitis exists.
      2) Abnormal neurologic exam.
      3) Child has been ill for several days.
      4) Recovery from febrile convulsion is slow.

    i. Electrolytes; cbc; glucose; Ca; Mg; skull x-rays are rarely helpful.

G. Shunt Malfunction

1. Anything that goes wrong with a patient with shunted hydrocephalus is due to a shunt problem until proved otherwise.
2. Signs and symptoms of acute obstruction include headache, irritability, lethargy, vomiting, bulging fontanelle, and behavior change. If present, evaluate as emergency.
3. Do not waste time pumping device; it may give misleading information. Do general/neurologic evaluation and call neurosurgeon for probable tap of pump device.
4. Most shunt infections occur within 2 mo of initial shunt placement.

H. Syncope

1. Syncope is a sudden, transient loss of consciousness (seconds to a minute or so) due to cerebral hypoperfusion or anoxia.
2. Important historical information includes:
   a. A complete description of the episode and antecedent events or patient's feelings (e.g., palpitation, dizziness, nausea, light headedness, etc.).
   b. A past history of similar events and their precipitating factors.
   c. Presence of tonic-clonic movements during the episode (R/O seizure).
   d. Cardiac symptoms (exertional dyspnea, palpitations).
   e. History of cardiac, CNS, pulmonary disease.
   f. Chronic medication use.
3. The PE is usually normal. It should be complete with special emphasis on cardiac exam (murmurs, arrhythmias, tachyarrhythmias) and the neurologic assessment, especially the patient's mental state and recollection of the event.
4. Causes of Syncope
   a. Vasovagal: Preceded by light-headedness, dizziness, diaphoresis, and pallor. This type of syncope may be preceded by physical discomfort, emotionally charged situations, or fright (as in seeing blood).
   b. Hysteria: The clue is that the patient is seemingly unconcerned about the event.
   c. Hyperventilation: Prolonged deep breathing intentionally or unintentionally during stress may lower pCO_2 enough to cause syncope. Other symptoms include chest tightness, weakness, and light-headedness.
   d. Breath-Holding: Usually precipitated by injury or anger. There may be cyanosis following crying or there may be pallor and collapse without antecedent crying.

e. Cardiac Lesions (aortic stenosis, pulmonic stenosis, truncus arteriosus, transposition of the great vessels, tetrology of Fallot, pulmonary hypertension, and carotid sinus syncope).

f. Cardiac Arrythmias (paroxysmal atrial tachycardia), atrioventricular block, paroxysmal ventricular fibrillation, long QT syndrome (episodes precipitated by physical or mental exertion), mitral valve prolapse (chest pain may also be present).

g. Postural hypotension.

h. Prolonged coughing.

i. Micturition.

j. Severe anemia.

k. Antihypertensives/antihistamines.

l. Cerebellar/brain stem tumors.

m. Hypoglycemia.

5. The history and PE guide the choice of laboratory tests.

a. Most individuals with a simple faint require no laboratory evaluation (except, perhaps, a dextrostix).

b. If there is a history of recurrent faints or "seizures" or if there are cardiac symptoms, an ECG is in order.

c. The patient's BP should be measured in supine, sitting, and standing positions.

6. Treatment is usually reassurance for most patients with syncope.

a. Patients with hyperventilation should be taught to breathe into a paper bag (increase $p\,CO_2$) during episodes.

b. Patients with hypoglycemia (transient) should be encouraged not to skip meals.

c. Those with chronic or recurrent hypoglycemia are managed as described in Ch. 5, C, "Hypoglycemia."

d. Individuals with postural hypotension should be reminded to go from a supine to standing position slowly.

  e. Correction of anemia, discontinuation of offending medications, and therapy of tumors should aid patients with these etiologies.

  f. Finally, individuals with cardiac processes should be managed in concert with a cardiologist.

I. Tics

1. A tic is a sudden, involuntary, repetitive, rapid, random, purposeless, highly stereotypic movement. The stereotypic nature differentiates it from chorea, myoclonus, athetosis, dystonia, and hemiballism. Other than their tics, affected children generally have normal exams.

2. a. Tics may be transient (duration in wk) or chronic (duration > 12 mo).

   b. They usually begin in the preschool or early school-age yrs.

   c. Tics may present singly or in groups. In addition, one tic might disappear only to be replaced by another.

   d. Tics typically wax and wane in severity. There is usually the ability to voluntarily suppress the tic for minutes to hrs.

3. a. Motor tics most commonly involve the head, face, and neck (examples are eye blinking, mouth twitching, head bobbing).

   b. Other children may develop hopping, jumping, skipping, and squatting.

4. a. Vocal tics are most commonly coughing, sniffing, and throat clearing.

   b. Other children may develop high-pitched cries, screams, barking, other animal noises, hiccuping, belching, echolalia, palilalia (repeating one's own words), or coprolalia (involuntary utterance of obscenities).

5. A subset of tic disorders is the Tourette's syndrome, which usually has its onset between 2 to 15 yrs.

a. The child has multiple muscle tics and multiple vocal tics.
b. Tics wax and wane over weeks, but the syndrome itself lasts for yrs or even a lifetime.
c. Familial clustering of affected individuals is common.
d. Some investigators believe that the syndrome may be precipitated or exacerbated by the use of methylphenidate (Ritalin) or Dexedrine.

6. No laboratory abnormalities have been detected in patients with tics or Tourette's syndrome.

7. Because of the side effects of the medications used to control tics, transient tics that are not socially objectionable should be permitted to spontaneously abate. Counseling of patient and parents is necessary.

8. a. For chronic tics and Tourette's syndrome, the mainstay of therapy is haloperidol (starting with 0.25-0.5 mg hs with 0.5 mg incremental increases every 4-5 days until the desired effect is achieved). The usual dose requirement is 2.0-2.5 mg/d. Side effects include lethargy, dysphoria, depression, and diminution of cognitive functioning. Extrapyramidal side effects (dystonia, tardive dyskinesia) have also been reported.
b. Counseling (psychotherapy) of patient and parents is necessary.

REFERENCES

Headache
1. Barabas G: Management of headaches in childhood. *Pediatr Ann* 1983; 12:806-13.
2. Olness K, MacDonald J: Recurrent headaches in children-Diagnosis and treatment. *Pediatr in Rev* 1987; 8:307-12.
3. Prensky A: Differentiating and Treating Pediatric Headaches. *Contemp Pediatr* 1984; 1:12-45.

Head Trauma
1. Dershewitz R et al: Treatment of children with post-traumatic transient loss of consciousness. *Pediatr* 1983; 72:602-7.
2. Leonidas JC, et al: Mild head trauma in children: When is a roentgenogram necessary? *Pediatr* 1982; 69:139-43.
3. Rosman NP: Pediatric emergencies - Managing acute head trauma. *Contemp Pediatr* 1986; 3:24-46.
4. Singer HS, Freeman JM: Head trauma for the pediatrician. *Pediatr* 1978; 62:819-25.
5. Steinbok P, et al: Management of simple depressed skull fractures in children. *J Neurosurg* 1987; 66:506-10.

Increased Intracranial Pressure
1. Griffith J, Brasfield J: Increased intracranial pressure. *Pediatr in Rev* 1981; 2:269-76.

CNS Infections
1. Congeni B: The treatment of bacterial meningitis. *Pediatr Ann* 1986; 15:456-60.
2. Gellis S, Kagan B (eds): *Current Pediatric Therapy - 12* Philadelphia: W.B. Saunders Co., 1986. pp. 62-3; 500-3; 590-1.
3. Klein J, et al: Report of the task force on diagnosis and management of meningitis. *Pediatr* 1986: 78 (suppl.).
4. McCracken G, et al: Consensus report - Antimicrobial therapy for bacterial meningitis in infants and children. *Pediatr Infect Dis* 1986; 6:501-5.
5. Wildin S, Chonmaitree T: The importance of the virology laboratory in the diagnosis and management of viral meningitis. *AJDC* 1987; 141:454-7.

Seizures

1. Barbosa E, Freeman J: Status epilepticus. *Pediatr in Rev* 1982; 4:185-9.
2. Consensus Development Panel: Febrile seizures - Long-term management of children with fever-associated seizures. *Pediatr in Rev* 1987; 2:209-12.
3. Dunn D: Anticonvulsants - When to start, what to use and when to stop. *Contemp Pediatr* 1986;' 3:50-68.
4. Gerger J, Berlinen B: The child with a "simple" febrile seizure. *AJDC* 198; 135:431-3.
5. Holmes G: Therapy of petit mal (absence) seizures. *Pediatr in Rev* 1982; 4:150-6.
6. Joffe A, et al: Which children with febrile seizures need lumbar puncture? *AJDC* 1983; 137:1153-6.
7. Rosman N, Oppenheimer E: Posttraumatic epilepsy. *Pediatr in Rev* 1982; 3;221-5.
8. Vining E, Freeman J: Status epilepticus. Pediatr Ann 1985; 14:764-70.
9. Vining E, Freeman J: Seizures which are not epilepsy. *Pediatr Ann* 1985; 14:711-23.
10. Vining E, Freeman J: Management of nonfebrile seizures. *Pediatr in Rev* 1986; 8:185-90.
11. Vining E, Freeman J: Special types of seizures. *Pediatr Ann* 1985; 14:747-62.
12. Wears R, et al: Which laboratory tests should be performed on children with apparent febrile convulsions? *Pediatr Emerg Care* 1986; 2:191-6.

Shunt Malfunction

1. Freeman JM, D'Souza B: Obstruction of CSF shunt. *Pediatr* 1979; 64:111-12.
2. Meirovitch J, et al: Cerebrospinal fluid shunt infections in children. *Pediatr Infec Dis* 1987; 6:921-4.
3. Yogev R: Cerebrospinal fluid shunt infections. *Pediatr Infec Dis* 1985; 4:113-8.

Syncope

1. Ruckman R: Cardiac causes of syncope. *Pediatr in Rev* 1987; 9:101-8.

Tics
1. Golden G: Tic Disorders in Childhood. *Pediatr in Rev* 1987; 8:229-33.
2. Golden G: Tics in Childhood. *Pediatr Ann* 1983; 12:821-4.
3. Shapiro A, Shapiro E: *Tics, Tourette Syndrome, and Other Movement Disorders.* New York: The Tourette Syndrome Association, 1980.

14

OPHTHALMOLOGY

A. Conjunctivitis: Lay term "Pink Eye"

1. Evaluation: Must differentiate conjunctivitis from more serious ocular inflammation (e.g., keratitis, iritis).

    a. Conjunctivitis: Diffuse redness of conjunctiva, associated with watery or purulent discharge, usually no photophobia, minimal pain, near normal vision, and normal pupillary reflexes. Etiologies: bacterial, viral, allergic, chemical.

    b. Keratitis: Acute inflammation of the cornea associated with extreme pain, tearing, and photophobia. Etiologies: Bacterial, viral, fungal, ultraviolet light (i.e., sunlamps). NOTE: Don't miss corneal ulcers or lacerations. Corneal injury may precede keratitis. Patient may have combined keratoconjunctivitis.

    c. Iritis: Red eye with little or no discharge, tearing, circumlimbal injection (not seen in conjunctivitis), photophobia, and pain. Pupil may be smaller and ± irregular. Vision may often be blurred.

    Refer to ophthalmologist if iritis or keratitis is suspected.

2. Etiology and Therapy of Conjunctivitis
   a. Neonate - Gram stain, Giemsa stain, bacterial, and chlamydial cultures are required.
      1) Chemical - secondary to AgNO3 drops; begins first day, usually clears in 24-48 hr. No treatment necessary.
      2) Gonococcal - begins on day 2-5, associated with purulent discharge, Gram stain shows G diplococci. Culture conjunctival scraping on Thayer-Martin.
         a) If Gram stain or culture confirms GC, admit for high-dose parenteral penicillin - 50,000 units/kg/d in 2 divided doses for 7 days, and saline eye flushes.
         b) GC rapidly penetrates cornea, therefore this dx requires immediate therapy.
         c) Both parents should be referred to public health authorities for epidemiologic case-finding and treatment.
      3) Chlamydial (Inclusion blenorrhea) - usually begins 3-30 days after birth. This is most common cause of conjunctivitis during the first two mo of life.
         a) Presumptive diagnosis can be made by noting cytoplasmic, basophilic inclusion bodies within epithelial cells on a Giemsa stained conjunctival smear. Only about half of cases are detected in this fashion.
         b) A more sensitive test, now available, is a <u>Chlamydia</u> fluorescent antibody slide test, which determines the presence of <u>Chlamydia</u> antigen.
         c) If the slide test results are negative, but <u>Chlamydia</u> is still strongly suspected, a <u>Chlamydia</u> culture can be sent for definitive diagnosis.
         d) Treatment consists of erythromycin 50 mg/kg/d in 4 divided doses po x 2 wk. There is no indication that topical therapy

provides additional benefit. Both parents should be treated if dx is made in neonate.

b. Allergic Conjunctivitis - characterized by itching, watery discharge, chemosis, periorbital edema, and other s/sx of allergy (allergic rhinitis, asthma, eczema).

1) Attempt to identify and eliminate the allergen from the patient's environment if possible (antibiotic eyedrops may be culprit),

2) Stop rubbing eyes,

3) Cold compresses,

4) Ophthalmic drops: Vasocon-A (contains vasconstrictor naphazoline), Muro-A, Naphcon-A (least painful), or Albalon-A, and antihistamine.

5) Systemic antihistamines and topical cromolyn may be helpful.

6) Extremely severe cases should be referred to an ophthalmologist for evaluation.

c. Bacterial - Gram stain purulent discharge, culture (not routinely necessary). Most common organisms are streptococci, pneumococci, staphylococci, and H. influenzae.

1) 10% sulfacetamide drops or erythromycin ophthalmic ointment qid x 1 wk.

2) Cases persisting despite treatment should be referred to an ophthalmologist.

N.B. Bacterial conjunctivitis under age of 2 yr is frequently associated with otitis media.

d. Viral - watery discharge plus inflammation.

1) Rx: nothing or sulfacetamide 10% ophthalmic drops to prevent bacterial superinfection.

2) Special N.B. on 2 viral etiologies that may involve both conjunctiva and cornea.

a) Epidemic keratoconjunctivitis (adenovirus type 8 and others).

Extremely contagious. Acute conjunctivitis with discomfort, preauricular adenopathy, corneal involvement with impaired vision several days later, associated with pain and photophobia. <u>Thorough</u> hand-washing and hygiene is imperative for family and medical personnel to minimize spread. Refer patient to an ophthalmologist. Often associated with pharyngitis (pharyngo-conjunctival fever).

b) Herpes simplex - may also present on eyelids and spread to conjunctiva and cornea. Significant in that blindness may result. <u>Topical steroids contraindicated.</u> Obtain culture and stain. Refer to an ophthalmologist. Viroptic (trifluorothymidine) is the drug of choice for topical therapy and Vira-A° ointment for lid disease.

B. Orbital Cellulitis

Infection of tissues behind orbital septum with involvement of retrobulbar structures (associated with proptosis, chemosis, limitation of eye movement, and possibly reduction of vision). Admit for urgent systemic antibiotic therapy. Bacterial etiology: <u>S. aureus,</u> Group A beta-hemolytic <u>Streptococcus,</u> or <u>H. influenzae.</u> Blood cultures are also indicated. Sinus evaluation with CT is indicated.

C. Periorbital Cellulitis

Cellulitis confined to eyelid (pre-septum). Most likely organisms are <u>S. aureus,</u> Group A beta-hemolytic <u>Streptococcus,</u> or <u>H. influenzae.</u> Requires admission for systemic therapy, although oral therapy may be adequate in mild cases.

N.B. There is a significant incidence of bacterial meningitis in children under 2 yr who have orbital or periorbital cellulitis. A spinal tap may be indicated, even in the absence of meningeal signs.

D. Stye (Hordeolum)

Infection (usually <u>S. aureus</u>) of one of the sebaceous glands along the lid margin that causes a small, red, tender swelling. Often suppurates and drains spontaneously.

1. Treatment consists of warm, moist compresses qid for 15 minutes each time, continuing until several days following clinical resolution.
2. A local ophthalmic ointment (Bacitracin, erythromycin) may be helpful.
3. Systemic antibiotics and I + D are rarely indicated.

E. Chalazion

Granulomatous infection of a meibomian gland (one of numerous sebaceous glands in the eyelid tarsus). It results in a slow-growing firm nodular swelling that most often points on the conjunctival aspect of the lid and usually causes little discomfort.

1. If it becomes secondarily infected, becoming inflamed and tender, apply warm, moist compresses qid for 15 minutes each time, continuing until one wk following clinical resolution.
2. If a chalazion persists for many months, it can be injected with a steroid (Triamcinolone) or incised with evacuation of its contents by an ophthalmologist.

F. Chemical Burns

Strong acids and especially strong alkali burns can be devastating.

1. Profuse irrigation of the eye with tap water should be instituted as soon as possible. If a family calls with such an injury, instruct them to irrigate the eye (being careful to retract both lids) immediately at home, and then proceed to the ER.
2. In the ER, apply 1-2 drops of a topical anesthetic, proparacaine HCL 0.5 (Ophthetic), to the eye to facilitate irrigation with an elevated bottle of normal saline and an IV tubing set - a convenient way

of providing a controlled and copious flow of irrigation fluid. Litmus paper touched to the conjunctival surface should register in the neutral range when irrigation is satisfactory.
3. Refer to ophthalmologist for assessment of extent of injury.

G. Corneal Abrasions and Foreign Bodies

Usually unilateral. Do fluorescein stain. Otherwise, refer to ophthalmologist.
1. A simple abrasion (no suspicion of a retained foreign body) is treated with a single application of 10% sulfacetamide ointment and tight eye patch x 24-48 hr.
2. Foreign bodies require prompt removal by an ophthalmologist, usually followed by a local antibiotic and patching.

H. Blunt Ocular Trauma ("Black Eye" or "Shiner")

Complete eye and fundus exam is indicated. Look for blow-out fracture of orbital floor, retinal detachment, hyphema, dislocated lens, traumatic iritis. Refer to ophthalmologist if there is any suspicion of the above complications.

I. Penetrating Ocular Trauma

Usually a perforation site can be seen with the naked eye. Another sign is distortion of the pupil. Apply a metal shield over the eye and do not put pressure on the eye.
Refer to ophthalmologist.
NOTE: In the initial evaluation of a patient with ocular trauma, do not forget to measure the visual acuity. Use the Snellen chart, Allen picture cards, or the "E" game. For children under 2 yr of age, observe the child's ability to use the damaged eye to reach for a small object.

J. Dacryostenosis

Congenital lacrimal duct obstruction. 80% of cases remit during first 6-9 mo. Characterized by excessive tearing in involved eye. May also have mild conjunctival injection with a purulent discharge.

1. Treatment involves massaging the lacrimal sac and sometimes treating with sulfacetamide drops or erythromycin ointment.
2. Probing of nasolacrimal duct is indicated if obstruction persists >9 mo.

K. Dacryocystitis

Delayed canalization of nasolacrimal duct with superimposed infection characterized by swelling, tenderness, and erythema below medial canthus.

1. Treat with IV or PO antibiotics against staphylococci, streptococci, and <u>H. influenzae.</u>
2. Warm compresses may speed resolution.
3. Once inflammation has diminished, lacrimal drainage system probing may be performed.

REFERENCES

1. Baker JD: Treatment of congenital nasolacrimal system obstruction. *J Pediatr Ophthalmol Strab* 1985; 22:34.
2. Bodor FF, Marchant CD, Shurin PA, et al: Bacterial etiology of conjunctivitis - otitis media syndrome. *Pediatr* 1985; 76:26-28.
3. Calhoun JH: Problems of the lacrimal system in children. *Pediatr Clin North Am* 1987; 34:1457-1465.
4. El-Mansoury J, Calhoun JH, Nelson LB, et al: Results of late probing for congenital nasolacrimal duct obstruction. *Ophthalmol* 1986; 93:1052.
5. Fisher MC: Conjunctivitis in children. *Pediatr Clin North Am* 1987; 34:1447-1456.
6. Friedlander MH, Okumoto M, Kelley J: Diagnosis of allergic conjunctivitis. *Arch Ophthalmol* 1984; 102:1198-1199.
7. Gigliotti F, Williams WT, Hayden FG: Etiology of acute conjunctivitis in children. *J Pediatr* 1981; 98:531-536.
8. Hammerschlag MR, Herrman JE, Cox P, et al: Enzyme immunoassay for diagnosis of neonatal Chlamydia conjunctivitis. *J Pediatr* 1985; 1076:741-743.
9. Knox DL: Uveitis. *Pediatr Clin N Am* 1987; 34:1467-1485.
10. Newell FW: *Ophthalmology Principles and Concepts*, 5th ed. C.V. Mosby Co., St. Louis, 1982.
11. Rettig PJ: Chlamydial infections in pediatrics: Diagnostic and therapeutic considerations. *Pediatr Inf Dis* 1986; 5:158-162.
12. Robb RM: Probing and irrigation for congenital nasolacrimal duct obstruction. *Arch Ophthalmol* 1986; 104:378.
13. Sandstron KI, Bell TA, Chandler JW, et al: Microbial causes of neonatal conjunctivitis. *J Pediatr* 1984; 105:706-711.
14. Siegel JD: Eye infections encountered by the pediatrician. *Pediatr Inf Dis* 1986; 5:741-748.

15

ORTHOPEDICS*

A. Bowlegs (Genu Varum)

    1. Infants are physiologically bowlegged due to their intrauterine position; however, this physiologic state corrects itself by 18-24 mo of age. The child's knee then develops a decided valgus before assuming the mild valgus of adulthood. (Fig 15-1).

*Patricia D. Fosarelli, M.D., with contributing author Paul D. Sponseller, M.D., Division of Pediatric Orthopedic Surgery, The Johns Hopkins Hospital.

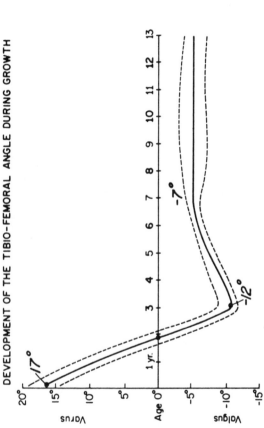

FIG 15-1. — "Bowed legs" and "knock knees." Note the broad variation with age. Varus corrects to neutral at approximately age 20 months, then recorrects to valgus by age 3 years, with slight valgus persisting to adulthood.

The degree of bowleggedness is appreciated on examination by bringing the medial malleoli together and measuring the distance between the two knees. In children with <u>physiologic</u> bowing, demonstrating the graph in Figure 15-1 is often reassuring to parents.

2. If correction has not begun by 24 mo or if the degree of bowing is >20°, serum calcium and phosphorus determination (R/O rickets) and radiographs of the lower limbs (R/O Blount's disease-see below) should be obtained. Physiologic bowing generally corrects by 2-3 yr of age. Some orthopedists recommend the use of splints, braces, or shoe bars.

3. Blount's disease (tibia vara) is the defective formation of the medial corner of the proximal tibial epiphysis (perhaps due to epiphyseal pressure caused by early or excessive weight bearing in a child with severe physiologic bowing). There are two variants: infantile and adolescent.

   a. The infantile variant occurs between 1 and 4 yr of age.

      1) Initially, these children are indistinguishable from infants with physiologic bowing.

      2) However, after 1-1/2–2 yr of age, their radiographs demonstrate angulation beneath the proximal epiphysis, (Fig 15-2) metaphyseal irregularities, proximal tibial breaking, and proximal epiphyseal wedging

      3) If the condition is detected between 18-24 mo of age, bracing with a valgus-producing brace may be effective.

      4) After the age of 3-4, surgery is usually indicated.

   b. The adolescent variant develops in obese children (>8 yr) or adolescents whose legs have been in slight varus; it is extremely uncommon and milder (<20° bowing) than the infantile variant. Previous epiphyseal injury may be pre-

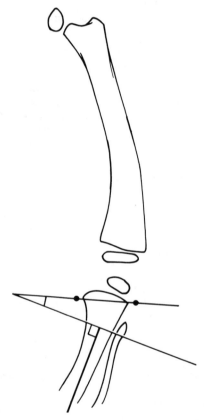

FIG 15-2. — In eary Blount's disease, the metaphyseal-diaphyseal angle is greater than 11°.

sent. Spontaneous regression may occur; however, progressive cases require surgery.

B. Congenital Dislocation of the Hip (CDH)

1. In CDH, the hip is dislocated as the femoral head is displaced from the hypoplastic acetabulum. Two frequent factors in its causation are liagamentous laxity and intrauterine breech position.
   The male-to-female ratio is 1:4-6. Genetic predisposition seems likely.

2. Infants with CDH usually (but not universally) have the folllowing:
   a. A positive Barlow's sign (hip is dislocatable by flexion, adduction, and axial pressure, Fig 15-3) and a positive Ortolani maneuver (as the flexed hip is slowly abducted, the femoral head shifts into the acetabulum producing a "clunk," Fig 15-4. One should perform these maneuvers on one hip at a time.

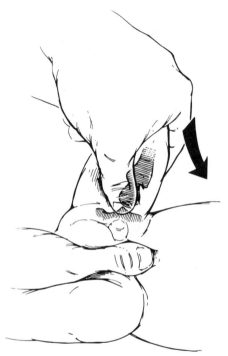

FIG 15-3. — Barlow's test: flexion-adduction and axial pressure elicit laxity or a "clunk" in an abnormal hip in a child up to 3 to 5 months old.

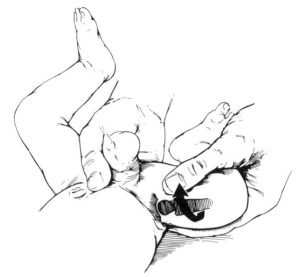

FIG 15-4. — Ortolani's test: the reduction of the dislocated hip by abduction in the flexed position. Examine only one hip at a time. Useful in children up to 3 to 5 months' of age.

      b. After age 3-6 mo when muscle contractures develop, the Barlow and Ortolani tests become negative. One then sees thigh fold asymmetry, leg length discrepancy (best seen when the infant is supine and the hips and knees are flexed to 90°), and limitation of hip abduction on the affected side (Fig 15-5).

   3. Older children with untreated CDH have a peculiar gait. Because the abductor muscles on the affected side are shortened and weakened, during the stance phase on the affected side, the opposite side of the pelvis drops. (Trendelenburg gait).

      Children with bilateral CDH have wide-set hips and a double Trendelenburg (waddling) gait.

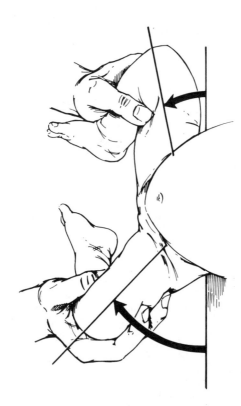

FIG 15-5. — In the older child with fixed dysplasia, in whom Barlow's and Ortolani's signs cannot be elicited, the main signs are limited abduction and apparent shortening.

4. Radiographs in the neonatal period are not necessarily diagnostic, but as the infant ages, they become so.

5. Successful treatment of CDH in the neonatal period is most reliably achieved by use of a Pavlik harness. This device holds the hips in reduction (hyperflexion (90°-100°) with no more than 60° of abduction) and permits diapering and cleaning of the infant.

   a. Extremes of flexion and abduction must be avoided, since they are associated with avascular necrosis and severe hip deformity.

   b. Infants aged 6-18 mo at diagnosis usually require traction, reduction under arthrographic control, and subsequent casting. Open surgery may be needed, if closed reduction is not possible. Avascular necrosis may still occur.

   c. Children 18-48 mo at diagnosis require surgery (muscle release, open reduction, and pelvic or femoral osteotomy) to obtain a stable hip. Avascular necrosis is a more frequent complication.

   d. Children older than 48 mo at diagnosis require more extensive surgical intervention. If their function is good, the risks and benefits of surgery fraught with so many potential complications must be carefully weighed.

C. In-toeing (Femoral Anteversion and Internal Tibial Torsion)

1. In evaluating the in-toeing child, three common conditions should be considered: Metatarsus adductus (section G), usually seen before age 1 1/2 yr; internal tibial torsion, ages 1 1/2-4 yr; and femoral anteversion, ages 3-8 yr. These can be sorted out by a systematic exam (Fig 15-6). The angle of the foot in walking should be noted (A). Then the child should be placed prone and checked for the thigh-foot angle (B), shape of foot (C), and hip rotation (D).

2. Tibial torsion measures 0°-20° (internal) at birth, and, with growth, derotation occurs until the adult configuration of 0°-40° (average 20°) of <u>external</u> tibial torsion is reached.

   a. The angle is measured as follows. The knee is flexed to 90°. The medial and lateral malleoli are palpated. In a neonate, the malleoli may be parallel, or the medial malleolus may lie behind the lateral malleolus. In the adult, the medial malleolus is forward of the lateral one.

   b. The angle may also be measured (with the child prone and the knee flexed) by estimating the angle between the foot axis and the thigh's long axis (Fig 15-6).

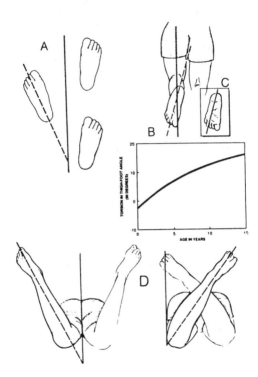

FIG 15-6. — Steps in assessing rotational abnormality. **A,** angle of the foot during walking should be observed. **B,** Bleck's line indicates the degree of forefoot adduction. Heel bisector should normally fall between second and third toe. **C,** thigh-foot angle reflects tibial torsion and becomes more external with age. Hip rotation of internal rotation **D,** is significantly greater than that of external rotation **E.** Anteversion or capsular tightness may be contributing to in-toeing.

3. Growth alone will correct the vast majority (99%) of cases of tibial torsion by age 3-4 yr.
   a. Correction may be accelerated by the use of night splints (tying heels of shoes together or Denis Browne bar).
   b. Shoe modifications are of no value.
   c. Rarely (1/1000) is surgery needed.
4. Excessive femoral anteversion occurs when the femoral neck is rotated forward or anteriorly more than usual from the femoral shaft (Fig 15-7). When the child stands, the leg rotates internally to accommodate the femoral head into the acetabulum. The underlying cause of excessive femoral anteversion is unknown. The child with femoral anteversion may present with internal rotation of the leg, flexible flat feet, and increased lumbar lordosis. On prone examination, internal rotation markedly exceeds external rotation (up to 90° vs < 30°); normally, external exceeds internal rotation.

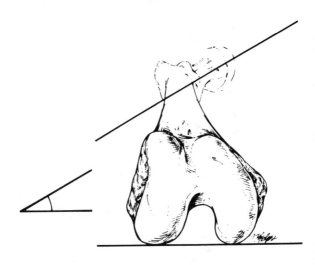

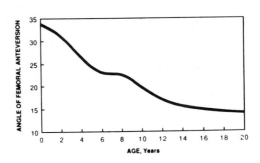

FIG 15-7. — Definition of anteversion and its normal variation.

5. Treatment consists of reassurance. By age 8 yr, 99% of all children with this finding experience resolution. Even if it persists, anteversion generally has no functional hindrance.
   a. For the 1% of children with severe deformity (internal hip rotation $\geq$ 80°, external rotation $\leq$ 15°, severe gait deformity, and absence of compensatory external tibial torsion), surgery will be necessary.
   b. Braces and cables have no influence on femoral anteversion.

D. Knock-Knees (Genu Valgum)

1. Most children are slightly knock-kneed at ages 3-5 yr; excessive knock-knee may develop in late childhood or adolescence. When the knees are touching, the medial malleoli cannot touch. The child may walk and run awkwardly, but he does not experience pain.
2. Genu valgum may be:
   a. Apparent (fat thighs, hypotonia, lax joints),
   b. Pathologic (paralytic disorders, JRA, rickets, trauma, bone, infections, Hubner's disease),
   c. Physiologic (idiopathic), accounting for the vast majority of the cases.
3. The diagnosis of idiopathic genu valgum should be made by a radiograph of the child's legs while he is standing (feet straight ahead); this is to exclude some of the pathologic causes of the disorder.
4. Idiopathic genu valgum resolves spontaneously with growth. Fewer than 1% of children who are affected will develop degenerative arthritis of the knee. With severe defects (i.e., >8 cm between medial malleoli), surgery may be needed; this is rare.

E. Legg-Calvé-Perthes Disease

1. Legg-Calvé-Perthes disease is avascular necrosis of the femoral head.

   a. The male-to-female ratio is 6:1.
   b. Etiology is unknown.
   c. Affected children are slightly shorter than peers and have delayed maturation.
   d. Routine childhood trauma may bring an asymptomatic child to attention.
2. There are five stages:
   a. Prenecrosis in which there is vascular compromise.
   b. Necrosis (3-6 mo) in which the affected section of bone dies with microfracture formation.
   c. Revascularization (6-12 mo) in which the dead bone is resorbed and replaced with cartilage.
   d. Reossification (18-36 mo) in which the deformed femoral head reossifies.
   e. Remodeling in which there is some improvement of the joint.
   f. The disease lasts 1-3 yr in most children.
3. The affected child has a limp, $\pm$ pain in the hip or thigh, and decreased hip motion (especially rotation and abduction).
4. The radiographic picture varies by the stage of the disease. There may be a widened joint space (growth failure), a lucent crescent under the femoral head margin, distortion of the femoral neck and head (shortened neck, flattened head), or loss of density in the metaphysis. A bone scan might quantify the amount of avascularity.
5. Treatment consists of restoring range of motion and maintaining the softened portion of the femur within the acetabular mold. This may require bed rest (often combined with Buck's traction if the range of motion is limited). If there is minimal involvement of the femoral head (<50%), or the child is under 6 yr, observation only is appropriate, checking for maintenance of range of motion. If there is >50% involvement or an older child, an abduction orthotic appliance or surgery may be employed to seat the femoral head within the acetabulum.

F. Limp

1. Limp can be painless or painful.
   a. Causes of <u>painless</u> limp include alteration in muscle tone and strength and joint function. Specifically, these include:
      1) Neurologic problems (flaccid paralysis, spasticity, ataxia, spinal diseases such as masses, herniated discs),
      2) Muscle disease (muscular dystrophy, arthrogryposis),
      3) Joint disorders (contractures, hyperextensible joints, congenital dislocated hip),
      4) Bone disorders (knock knees, leg length discrepancies, Blount's disease, tibial torsion, slipped capital femoral epiphysis, coxa vara, epiphyseal dysplasias, spondylolisthesis),
      5) Hysteria or mimicry. Generally, painless limps are insidious in onset. The child is not acutely ill. The etiology is usually apparent from the PE, which must include a careful neurologic assessment to R/O intraspinal disorders.
   b. Causes of <u>painful</u> limp include:
      1) Trauma (local-especially foot lesions, ligamentous strains and sprains, tendonitis, tendon tears, muscle bruises, fractures, injections, or patellar subluxation in adolescent girls).
      2) Infections (septic joint, osteomyelitis, pyomyositis, intervertebral disc inflammation or infection, epidural abscess),
      3) Intra-abdominal processes (appendicitis, retroperitoneal masses, iliac adenitis),
      4) Inflammatory disorders (toxic synovitis, rheumatic fever, JRA, SLE, and other collagen-vascular disorders),
      5) Aseptic necrosis and osteochondritis (Legg-Calvé-Perthes, Osgood-Schlatter, chondromalacia patellae, osteochondritis dissecans),

6) Neoplasms (leukemia, malignant and benign bone tumors),

7) Hematologic disorders (hemophilia with hemarthrosis, SS disease [hand-foot syndrome], phlebitis, scurvy).

8) Miscellaneous (Henoch-Schönlein purpura, serum sickness, and inflammatory bowel diseases).

2. The painful limp may have an acute or gradual onset; the child may be febrile (infectious processes) or may be afebrile. Depending on the etiology, the child may have GI symptoms or dermatologic findings.

a. The history should address all these issues with particular emphasis on the limp's onset, progression, duration, aggravating factors, and measures to relieve the pain.

b. Any other symptoms of illness should be elicited; the presence of chronic conditions, medication use, previous orthopedic injury, or surgery should be revealed.

c. Don't forget child abuse.

3. The child's PE should be complete.

a. The affected limb's appearance, joints, symmetry with its mate, and range of motion (active and passive) should be assessed.

b. The limbs should be systematically palpated for tenderness as a minor buckle fracture might be subtle. Most common areas are distal tibia and calcaneus. Palpation is also a good way to localize a possible osteomyelitis.

c. The skin and other joints should be carefully examined.

d. To R/O an abdominal process, a meticulous abdominal and rectal exam must be performed.

4. Laboratory tests are dictated by the history and physical findings.

a. A radiograph of the entire limb may be useful to identify and localize the problem.

b. If the child appears ill, a cbc with diff, ESR, and blood culture are in order.

c. A suspicious joint neeeds to be tapped. If abuse is suspected, a radiographic trauma series may be in order.

5. Treatment of limp is directed at the underlying disorder, most of which have been discussed elsewhere.

G. Metatarsus Adductus

1. In metatarsus adductus, the bones of the forefoot are deviated medially on the bones of the midfoot at the tarso-metatarsal joint. It is most prominent at the first joint. The sole of the foot is laterally convex and medially concave; the fifth metatarsal may be subject to excessive weight-bearing forces. When the child stands, his hindfoot may be in a valgus position.

   Metatarsus adductus may be supple or fixed. Genetic and intrauterine forces may play roles in its genesis.

2. Supple metatarsus adductus implies that the deviation is easily correctible with passive manipulation of the foot.

   a. Children with this variant usually require either no treatment or simple stretching exercises.

   b. At diaper changes, the parent holds the heel in one hand and gently exerts laterally-directed pressure against the first metatarsal with the other hand.

   c. Straight-last or outflare shoes, worn day and night, may also be of benefit.

3. Children with rigid metatarsus adductus (passive correction impossible) often will not correct spontaneously. They require serial cast or brace correction; if begun in the first through sixth mos of life, correction usually occurs in 1-2 mo. Serial casting may be effective up to 1 to 2 yr of age but is ineffective after 2 yr.

After the deformity has been corrected by the casts, holding casts or straight-last/outflare shoes are used until there is no chance of recurrence. Children older than 2 yr usually require surgery to correct their defects, if symptomatic.

H. Osgood-Schlatter Disease

1. Osgood-Schlatter disease consists of a painful enlargement of the tibial tuberosity due to vigorous quadriceps pull in a growing child. The inflammation at the patellar tendon insertion accounts for the symptoms of pain below the kneecap especially during physical acitivity or kneeling.

   The examiner can elicit this pain by pressing on the tibial tuberosity at the patellar tendon insertion. If the presentation is classic, a radiograph is unnecessary. (The radiograph shows an irregular, prominent tubercle; ossicles may be present in the tendon).

2. The disease is self-limited; symptoms will cease when the proximal tibial epiphysis closes (age 14-16).

   a. Mild cases can be managed by rest, quadriceps and hamstring stretching, restriction of activity, NSAIDs, and ice packs. After the pain subsides, activity can be resumed gradually.

   b. In more severe cases, crutches, knee immobilization, or casting may be necessary.

I. Scoliosis

1. Scoliosis is a lateral curvature of the spine. Most cases are idiopathic, but there are congenital and neuromuscular causes.

   a. Girls are more frequently affected than boys.

   b. The usual onset is after 9-10 yr for girls and after 11-12 yr for boys.

2. Screening for scoliosis should begin at 6-7 yr of age (Fig 15-8).

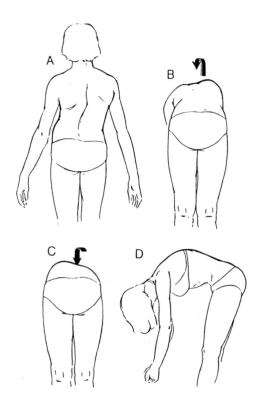

FIG 15-8. — Screening for spinal deformities. **A,** scoliosis may be demonstrated by subtle or striking elevation of one shoulder, trunk shift, and waistline asymmetry. **B,** forward bending with the hands clasped and the knees straight might reveal a thoracic prominence on the convex side, even if the standing exam appears normal. **C,** further forward bending will show any lumbar curve (usually opposite of thoracic curve). **D,** always look from side to see a focal kyphosis.

a. Look at the standing child from behind for asymmetry of the arm/trunk angles, shoulder lines, and flank creases.

b. Place your hands on the iliac crests to detect differences in leg lengths.

c. Have the patient bend at the waist as he/she extends the arms in front with palms together (a diving position). As the child bends to touch the toes, observe the horizontal plane of each set of vertebrae to determine on which side an elevation occurs. (N.B. The elevation is on the convex side of the curve, and the depression is on the concave side).

d. Observe the patient from the side during the bending test to determine if there is kyphosis (an abnormal angling of the spine rather than its rounded contour).

3. Worsening of scoliotic curves is associated with:

a. Younger age (<12 yr) at diagnosis, especially if the curve is severe.

b. Location of the curve, with thoracic and thoracolumbar the most likely to progress.

c. Severity of the curve, with those of 30°-40° and more the most likely to progress.

d. Skeletal immaturity, as measured by the ossification of the iliac apophysis.

e. Sex: small curves in boys are much less likely to progress.

4. Refer patient for radiographs or an orthopedic consult, if the angle of trunk rotation (i.e., the angle between the horizontal plane and a plane across the posterior trunk at the point(s) of <u>maximum</u> deformity) is greater than 5°, or if the vertebral angulation (Cobb measurement) is over 20-25°.

If a smaller curve is present, the child should still be followed by bend test or x-ray until growth ceases.

J. Slipped Capital Femoral Epiphysis (SCFE)

1. SCFE is an abrupt or gradual displacement of the proximal femoral epiphysis on the femoral neck.
   a. The male-to-female ratio is 2-3:1, and it most commonly occurs in preadolescence or adolescence.
   b. The cause is unknown, but the following factors have been implicated: Obesity, growth spurt, hormonal factors, an intrinsically defective growth plate, genetic predisposition, and trauma.

2. The child may present acutely with a painful limp and pain in the groin, thigh, or knee. Hip motion is painful and limited (especially abduction and internal rotation). Flexing the involved hip causes external rotation.
   Alternatively, the child may present with a gradual onset of intermittent pain and limping.

3. The radiographs of SCFE may show a widened growth plate of the proximal femur on the affected side.
   a. In true cases, the film will demonstrate the altered position of the head and neck.
   b. The medial and posterior displacement of the femoral head with apparent loss of height can be seen, especially by drawing a line up along the lateral aspect of the femoral neck.
   c. Since many slips are posterior, a cross-table lateral film is mandatory.

4. Treatment of SCFE is directed toward preventing further slippage, avascular necrosis, premature degenerative arthritis, and further gait deterioration.
   a. The patient with suspected SCFE should be forbidden to walk.
   b. Fixation of the slip may be achieved through screw insertion or open-bone-graft epiphysiodesis.

K. Subluxed Radial Head

1. The radial head temporarily loses contact with the capitellum, and the annular ligament surrounding the radial neck becomes partially interposed between joint surfaces (Fig 15-9).

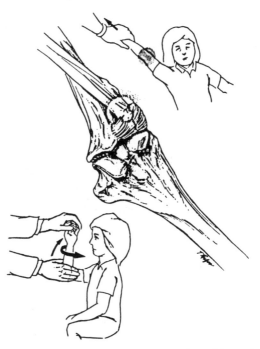

FIG 15-9. — "Pulled" or "nursemaid's" elbow is a partial tear of the annular ligament of the radial head. It can be reduced by flexion and supination.

     a. This series of events occurs when a young child's forearm or wrist is jerked with longitudinal and pronational forces.

     b. The child holds his arm in extension and actively resists attempts to flex it.

     c. Radiographs are normal.

2. Treatment consists of hypersupination of the forearm with the elbow held in flexion; once the child's ligament is released, he begins to use his arm again. Some orthopedists recommend a posterior splint for 10 days to allow healing of the ligament, especially if the subluxation is recurrent.

Parents and siblings should be educated about the mechanism of injury and discouraged from jerking the arm.

L. Torticollis

1. Torticollis (wryneck, tilted neck) may be congenital (vertebral anomalies, tumors, intrauterine malposition, birth trauma) or acquired (vertebral column or spinal tumors; inflammatory, such as cervical adenitis or intervertebral discitis; or traumatic, such as cervical subluxation or neck muscle strain).

The most common cause is neck muscle strain acquired during play, participation in sports, or sleeping in an awkward position.

2. The child presents with his head tilted toward the affected side. The sternocleidomastoid muscle is shortened due to muscle spasm.

     a. Because torticollis may be secondary to subluxation or dislocation of the facets of the atlantoaxial joint, anteroposterior, lateral, and openmouth odontoid radiographs should be obtained if suspicion is high.

     b. Children with torticollis and neurologic deficits should have their necks stabilized and neurosurgical consultation.

3. Treatment of torticollis due to neck strain con-

sists of warm soaks, analgesics, mild anti-inflammatory agents, and a soft cervical collar.

Treatment of torticollis due to atlanto-axial subluxation consists of rest and cervical traction; a soft collar may provide relief after reduction. Surgery is rarely necessary.

M. Transient Synovitis

1. Toxic or transient synovitis is an acute inflammation of the hip in a child 2-12 yr of age. Boys are more frequently affected than girls. The cause is unknown.

2. The child may present with a limp; groin, hip, thigh, and knee pain are also reported. The limp is characterized by a shortened stance on the affected side, with guarding or spasm of the muscles around the hip joint. Severely affected children may refuse to walk at all. All symptoms are of an acute onset.

   On examination, the child has limited active and passive range of motion at the hip due to muscle guarding.

3. If the child is febrile or if there is suspicion that he has a septic joint, certain laboratory tests are indicated. However, in toxic synovitis, the cbc with diff and ESR will be normal or only mildly elevated; so, too, is the hip radiograph (although the soft tissue planes around the hip may be distorted).

   If, by exam and cbc/ESR, a septic hip cannot be ruled out, aspiration of the joint under fluoroscopy should be performed. The joint fluid is always sterile, as opposed to the fluid from a septic joint, which has wbc and may have organisms on Gram-stain.

4. Hospitalization may be necessary if the child has a high fever or severe symptoms.

   a. If the child is not hospitalized, serial examinations of the hip should be done every few days (as synovitis may be the herald of osteomyelitis,

neoplasm, Legg-Calvé-Perthes disease, or SCFE.
   b. Toxic synovitis usually resolves in 3-5 d; prolongation of symptoms should prompt reconsideration of the diagnosis.
   c. Treatment consists of rest, analgesics, and restricted activity; severely affected patients may benefit from light skin traction.

REFERENCES

Bowlegs
1. McDade W: Bow legs and Knock Knees. *PCNA* 1977; 24:825-39.
2. Renshaw T: *Pediatric Orthopedics*. Phildelphia: W.B. Saunders Co., 1986, pp. 101-2.
3. Scoles P: *Pediatric Orthopedics in Clinical Practice*. Chicago: Year Book Medical Publishers, 1982. pp. 90-2.
4. Staheli L: Torsional Deformity. PCNA 1977; 24:799-811.

Congenital Hip Dislocation
1. Renshaw T: *Pediatric Orthopedics*. Philadelphia: W.B. Saunders Co., 1986, pp. 63-71.
2. Scoles P: *Pediatric Orthopedics in Clinical Practice*. Chicago: Year Book Medical Publishers, 1982. pp. 123-39.
3. Sherk H, et al: Congenital dislocation of the hip. *Clin Pediatr* 1981; 20:513-20.
4. Staheli L: Congenital hip dislocation. *Perinatal Care*. 1978; 2:14-17.

In-Toeing
1. Connolly J, et al: Pigeon-toes and flat feet. *PCNA* 1970; 17:291-307.
2. Eilert R, et al: Foot Care for the Very Young Patient. *Patient Care* 1979; 108-140.
3. Renshaw T: *Pediatric Orthopedics*. Philadelphia: W.B. Saunders Co., 1986. pp. 96-9.
4. Rosman M: When parents ask about in-toeing. *Contemp Pediatr* 1987; 3:116-22.
5. Scoles P: *Pediatric Orthopedics in Clinical Practice*. Chicago: Year Book Medical Publishers, 1982. pp. 93-98.

Knock-Knees
1. McDade W: Bow legs and Knock Knees. *PCNA* 1977; 24:825-39.
2. Renshaw T: *Pediatric Orthopedics*. Philadelphia: W.B. Saunders Co., 1986. p. 100.

Legg-Calvé-Perthes Disease
1. Bunnell W: Legg-Calvé-Perthes disease. *Pediatr in Rev* 1986; 7:299-304.
2. Griffiths H: Etiology, pathogenesis, and early diagnosis of ischemic necrosis of the hip. *JAMA* 1981; 246:2615-17.

3. Renshaw T: *Pediatric Orthopedics*. Philadelphia: W.B. Saunders Co., 1986. pp. 77-83.
4. Scoles P: *Pediatric Orthopedics in Clinical Practice*. Chicago: Year Book Medical Publishers, 1982. pp. 161-171.
5. Thompson G, et al: *Legg-Calvé-Perthes Disease* (CIBA Clinical Symposia). Vol. 38, 1986.

Limp
1. Hensinger R: Limp. *PCNA* 1977; 24:723-30.
2. Kaye J: Roentgenographic Evaluation of Children with Acute Onset of Limp. *Ped Annals* 1976; 11-29.
3. Singer J: The cause of gait disturbance in 425 pediatric patients. *Pediatr Emerg Care* 1985; 1:7-10.
4. Tunnessen W: *Signs and Symptoms in Pediatrics*. Philadelphia: J.B. Lippincott Co., 1983. pp. 460-5.

Metatarsus Adductus
1. McDade W: Bow legs and knock knees. *PCNA* 1977; 24:825-39.
2. Renshaw T: *Pediatric Orthopedics*. Philadelphia: W.B. Saunders Co., 1986. pp. 123-4.
3. Rosman M: When parents ask about in-toeing. *Contemp Pediatr* 1987; 3:116-22.
4. Scoles P: *Pediatric Orthopedics in Clinical Practice*. Chicago: Year Book Medical Publishers, 1982. pp. 103-113.
5. Staheli L: Torsional deformity. *PCNA* 1977; 24:799-811.

Osgood-Schlatter Disease
1. Mital M, Matza R: Osgood-Schlatter Disease. *The Physician and Sports Medicine* 1977; 60-73.
2. Scoles P: *Pediatric Orthopedics in Clinical Practice*. Chicago: Year Book Medical Publishers, 1982. p. 120.

Scoliosis
1. Berweick D: Scoliosis screening. *Pediatr in Rev* 1984; 5:238-47.
2. Bunnell W: Are you over-referring scoliosis? *Contemp Pediatr* 1985; 1:64-76.
3. Renshaw T: *Pediatric Orthopedics*. Philadelphia: W.B. Saunders Co., 1986. pp. 5-6, 42-9.
4. Scoles P: *Pediatric Orthopedics in Clinical Practice*. Chicago: Year Book Medical Publishers, 1982. pp. 190-211.

SCFE
1. Renshaw T: *Pediatric Orthopedics*. Philadelphia: W.B. Saunders Co., 1986. pp. 83-6.
2. Scoles P: *Pediatric Orthopedics in Clinical Practice*. Chicago: Year Book Medical Publishers, 1982. pp. 171-77.

Subluxed Radial Head
1. Nichols H: Nursemaid's elbow-Reducing it to simple terms. *Contemp Pediatr* 1988; 3:50-7.
2. Quan L, Marcuse E: The epidemiology and treatment of radial head subluxation. *AJDC* 1985; 139:1194-7.
3. Renshaw T: *Pediatric Orthopedics*. Philadelphia: W.B. Saunders Co., 1986. p. 24.

Torticollis
1. Renshaw T: *Pediatric Orthopedics*. Philadelphia: W.B. Saunders Co., 1986. pp. 41-2.
2. Scoles P: *Pediatric Orthopedics in Clinical Practice*. Chicago: Year Book Medical Publishers, 1982. pp. 218-23.

Transient Synovitis
1. Haueisen D, et al: The characterization of "Transient Synovitis of the Hip" in children. *J Pediatr Orthop* 1986; 6:11.
2. Renshaw T: *Pediatric Orthopedics*. Philadelphia: W.B. Saunders Co., 1986. pp. 87-8.
3. Scoles P: *Pediatric Orthopedics in Clinical Practice*. Chicago: Year Book Medical Publishers, 1982. pp. 159-161.

16

OTOLARYNGOLOGY

A. Allergic Rhinitis

Commonest cause of chronic nasal congestion in children.

1. Etiology
   a. In young children causes are usually perennial: dust mite, molds, and animal dander.
   b. In older children (>4 yr) often seasonal: tree/grass pollens in spring, ragweed in fall. Environmental history is crucial - PLAY DETECTIVE!
   c. Symptoms often aggravated by smoking, pollutants, temperature, and humidity changes.
2. Signs and Symptoms
   a. Triad of sneezing, nasal congestion, watery discharge.
   b. "Allergic salute," "allergic shiners," mouth-breathing.
   c. PE - pale, bluish, boggy mucosa, enlarged turbinates; with perennial Sx may see otitis, nasal speech, snoring, malaise, epistaxis.
3. Differential Dx
   a. Foreign body - unilateral purulent discharge with odor.
   b. Anatomic - septal deviation.

  c. Chronic infection - sinusitis, adenoiditis (purulent nasal discharge, low grade fever, malaise, anorexia).

  d. Chronic use of topical agents (rhinitis medicamentosum).

  e. Vasomotor (non-allergic, non-infectious): thin discharge, unimpressive, neg Hx for allergy, neg skin tests.

   1) Eosinophilic

   2) Non-eosinophilic

 4. Diagnostic Aids

  a. Hansel stain of nasal secretions - VERY HELP-FUL.

Staining of Nasal Secretions

  1) Blow nose into plastic or wax paper wrap.

  2) Spread on glass slide and dry overnight.

  3) Stain for 30 s with Hansel stain.

  4) Add distilled water for 30 s.

  5) Wash with water.

  6) Decolorize with methanol or 95% ethyl alcohol.

  7) Dry and examine under oil.

   >10% EOS suggests allergy. Sheets of polys and bacteria suggest bacterial infection.

---

  b. Skin tests for patients not responding to usual Rx.

  c. Sinus x-rays to R/O bacterial infection.

 5. Treatment

  a. Avoidance of suspected allergens.

  b. Antihistamines: Start low and increase to tolerance or effect (Terfenadine {Seldane} associated with less drowsiness.

  c. Oral decongestants.

  d. Topical agents

   1) Cromolyn - only for prophylaxis.

2) Steroids (beconase, nasilide, funisilide) not well absorbed from mucosa. May be irritating.
   e. Immunotherapy for treatment failures, especially when clinical history and skin tests concur.

B. Epistaxis

Peak age 4-10yr; boys > girls. Usually from anterior portion of nasal septum.
1. Etiology
   a. Young children - trauma, inflammation.
   b. Older children - dryness, crusting, "picking."
      N.B. In teenage girls may be associated with menses.
      Teenage boys - think of angiofibroma.
   c. Blood dyscrasia/clotting abnormalities rare but need to consider with chronic/recurrent episodes.
2. Diagnosis
   a. Careful exam to identify bleeding point.
   b. cbc/clotting studies with recurrent episodes.
3. Management
   a. Compression of anterior nasal septum ~ 10 minutes with gauze soaked with 1: 1000 epinephrine may be helpful.
   b. With persistent bleeding - silver nitrate cautery and/or packing (gel foam, petrolatum gauze).
   c. If bleeding is profuse or site not located, get help from ENT.
   d. In cases due to dryness/crusting/"picking," humidification, and local petrolatum can be helpful.

C. Foreign Bodies

1. Ear
   Etiology: Can be almost anything. At Johns Hopkins, roaches, paper, toy parts, earring parts, hair beads, erasers occur in that order.

Presentation: Pain, decreased hearing, discharge, "digging at ear."

Management: 90% can be removed in office/ER with simple equipment. Parents should be cautioned against trying to remove objects at home. Cooperation is essential. Sedation and topical anesthesia (2% lidocaine spray) may be helpful.

 a. If object does not completely occlude canal, use ear loop, curette (friable objects), or forceps.

 b. For rounded or softer non-vegetable objects (if TM intact), irrigate with water-pik and tepid water.

 c. Two choices for insects

  1) Fill ear canal with mineral oil, then irrigate.

  2) Irrigate ear canal with 2% lidocaine; this will usually cause varmit to flee but may be associated with vertigo. If the canal is swollen, there is significant bleeding, or the FB cannot be <u>easily</u> removed - call for help (spelled ENT)!

N.B. A new hazard is the alkaline button battery. These can produce rapid tissue destruction on contact with moist tissue and can lead to perforation of TM, destruction of ossicles, and ulceration of local tissues. These should be removed by ENT, either under sedation or general anesthesia.

2. Nose

Etiology: Hair beads, toy parts, paper, food, crayons, erasers.

Presentation: Pain, foul odor, discharge, bleeding. Can sometimes present as <u>generalized</u> body odor. Unilateral purulent and/or malodorous nasal discharge is <u>always</u> suggestive of a foreign body.

Management: Most can be handled in the office/ER with simple equipment. Parents should be cautioned against trying to remove objects at home. Cooperation, topical anesthesia (2% lidocaine), and vasoconstriction are all helpful. Important not to push objects into the nasopharynx where it can be aspirated by struggling child.

    a. Most objects can be removed by small hook, loop, forceps, or nasal suction.

    b. Cooperative child can be asked to apply positive pressure through his/her nose.

    c. Unesthetic but effective technique is to occlude non-obstructed nostril with digital pressure and blow into patient's mouth (with tight seal). This should be reserved for relatives and close friends.

    d. Button batteries can rapidly cause tissue damage - need to be removed quickly.

3. Upper Airway

    a. Laryngotracheal

    Presentation: Dyspnea, cough, stridor, and wheezing.A choking episode is observed in 90% of cases. Commonly confused with croup. FB should always be considered in differential diagnosis of croup, especially in absence of URI symptoms.

    Diagnosis: Lateral neck and high KV films of the airway may be helpful. Chest x-ray is usually normal. If suspicious of foreign body in upper airway - refer to ENT for endoscopy.

    Mangement: Removal via rigid endoscope.

    b. Cricopharyngeal

    Presentation: Dysphagia, excessive salivation, pain in throat, FB sensation. Tenderness on palpation over trachea. N.B. There may be no clinical findings in many of these cases.

    Diagnosis: Intra-oral exam, indirect laryngoscopy, and high KV of the airway may be helpful. A negative x-ray is not helpful.

    Mangement: Removal via rigid endoscope.

4. Esophagus

Etiology: Mostly coins, followed by safety pins, straight pins, and hairpins.

Presentation: Usually lodge in the upper 1/3 of the esophagus. Symptoms include chest and abdominal pain, coughing, choking, vomiting, and drooling. Metallic foreign bodies are easily diagnosed by x-ray.

Management: Esophageal foreign bodies require prompt removal.

a. Sharp objects should be removed via rigid bronchoscope under general anesthesia.

b. Smooth objects (coins) can be removed by:
   1) Foley catheter under fluoroscopy.
   2) Fiberoptic endoscope.

N.B. If Foley catheter is used, be prepared for possibility of aspiration and airway obstruction. Person experienced in pediatric airway maintenance should be available.

Always get a plain film just prior to procedure to verify that object is still present.

c. The majority of FBs which reach the stomach will eventually pass through the GI tract. Endoscopic removal indicated only if object remains in the stomach >14 days.

D. Hoarseness

1. Acute - sudden voice change lasting only a few days.
   a. Etiology: Acute inflammation of cords secondary to viral URI, vocal abuse such as screaming, shouting, singing.
   b. Treatment: Humidification, gargles, hot/cold liquids.

2. Chronic - voice change lasting several wk.
   a. Etiology: Vocal abuse/misuse-"screamer's nodes" (nodules on vocal cords) tumors (rare) such as laryngeal papillomas.
   b. Treatment: Symptomatic; speech therapy, endoscopic removal of nodules is rarely indicated.
      Laryngoscopy indicated if hoarseness persists beyond a few wk, is recurrent, or is accompanied by stridor or increased respiratory effort.

E. Otitis (Acute, Serous, Externa)

1. Acute Otitis Media
   a. Symptoms: Ear pain, pulling at ear. May present with nonspecific findings of $\pm$ fever, irritability, vomiting, and diarrhea. Often associated with URI.
   b. Signs: Hallmark is tympanic immobility.
      1) Erythema of TM (Crying alone may cause mild injection of TM).
      2) Poor, absent, distorted landmarks: dull, bulging, distorted light reflex.
      3) Asymmetry of appearance of TMs.
   c. Etiology
      <3 months: consider usual pathogens <u>(S. pneumoniae, H. influenzae, B. catarrhalis)</u> plus gram negative organisms, <u>S. aureus</u> and <u>C. trachomatis.</u>
      >3 months: 30% <u>S. pneumoniae,</u> 20% <u>H. influenzae,</u> 20% <u>B. catarrhalis,</u> remainder due to a variety of bacteria, viruses, (?) mycoplasma. 30% of <u>H. influenzae</u> strains and 75% of <u>B. catarrhalis</u> strains isolated from middle ear fluid are beta-lactamase producers.
   d. Treatment
      1) Neonatal Otitis: Consider admission because of risk of sepsis, meningitis. May warrant tympanocentesis along with full sepsis W/U. Broad-spectrum IV antibiotic coverage is indicated.
      2) >3 months: Several approaches to therapy.
         a) Amoxicillin + clavulanate potassium (40 mg/kg/d ÷ tid x 10d), cefaclor (Ceclor) (40 mg/kg/d ÷ tid x 10d) or erythromycin ethylsuccinate and sulfisoxazole (Pediazole) (50 mg/kg/d erythromycin ÷ qid x 10d).
                          OR
         b) Amoxicillin (40 mg/kg/d ÷ tid x 10d); if no response within 48 hr, switch to one of the above regimens or trimethoprim-sul-

famethoxazole (Bactrim, Septra) (8 mg/kg/d TMP, 40 mg/kg/d SMZ + bid x 10d).

c) If allergy to penicillin, use Pediazole or TMP-SMZ.

e. Patient should note improvement in 48 hr. If no improvement, consider poor compliance, resistant organism, or viral etiology.

f. Antihistamines and decongestants: no evidence of efficacy.

g. Analgesics/Antipyretics: prn for fever, pain. Auralgan Otic Drops (antipyrine, benzocaine, glycerin) local anesthetic for canal/TM. Do not use if TM has perforated or there is a discharge in canal.

h. Bullous myringitis: Bullae on TM. Often hemorrhagic. Painful. Etiologies include bacterial or viral. Infrequently, mycoplasma. Treat as acute bacterial otitis media.

i. Prophylaxis of recurrent OM (> 3 episodes in 5 mo): sulfisoxazole (500 mg bid) or amoxicillin (20 mg/kg hs) x 6 mo. If this fails, referral to ENT is indicated for probable tympanostomy tube placement. Role of adenoidectomy is not clearly defined but may be indicated if there is evidence of upper airway obstruction.

j. In patient with recurrent otitis, evaluate for underlying problem, i. e., allergy, immune defect, chronic sinusitis, anatomic defect in upper airway.

2. Serous Otitis Media (secretory otitis, middle ear effusion).

All children with acute otitis media should be rechecked after 10-day course of antibiotic therapy. Middle ear effusion will be present in 50% of pt at 2 wk F/U; 20% at 8 wk F/U, and 5-10% at 12 wk F/U.

Middle ear effusion may be picked up as incidental finding in asymptomatic pt. In ~ 50% of these patients, pathogenic bacteria will be recovered from middle ear fluid.

May also be associated with allergy, eustachian tube dysfunction, smoking in household.

a. Dx. - dull, gray, thickened, retracted TM with decreased mobility; $\pm$ air fluid levels behind TM, abnormal tympanogram.

b. Natural history - most cases appear to resolve spontaneously over several wk to mo but may be associated with significant hearing loss.

c. Treatment

1) Antibiotics: if pt has not been Rx with antibiotics, 10-14d course is indicated. If pt has been Rx, 10-14d course with a different agent is indicated.

2) Decongestants and antihistamines: no evidence of efficacy.

3) Steroids: no evidence that steroid (PO or intranasal) alone is effective, but 1 wk course of PO prednisone plus 2-4 wk course of antibiotic may be effective. Probably indicated before ENT referral.

4) If middle ear effusion persists >3 mo in spite of Rx with antibiotic and (?) prednisone, referral to ENT is indicated for myringotomy and tympanostomy tube placement.

5) The role of adenoidectomy is not clearly defined but may be indicated in patient with upper airway obstruction.

N.B. In infants with recurrent OM or middle ear effusion, bottle propping and feeding in the recumbent position should be discouraged.

3. Otitis Externa

a. Inflammation of skin lining auditory canal, often secondary to trauma (from Q-tips, bobbi pins, etc.) and/or infection. Also known as "swimmer's ear."

b. Symptoms: Pain on pulling the pinna or tragus, itching, + discharge.

    c. Signs: Edematous, erythematous auditory canal with discharge.

    d. Treatment

       1) Steroid-antibiotic drops (Cortisporin) 2-4 drops in affected ear qid x 5-7 days. Use Cortisporin suspension, not solution, if PE tubes are in place. Cortisporin solution causes pain on contact with middle ear. A cotton wick can be inserted in the auditory canal and moistened with Cortisporin q 4h.

       2) Avoid swimming until problem resolves.

  4. Chronic Otitis

  Chronic suppurative otitis media in which ear discharge is present in a child with a perforated TM or a tympanostomy tube requires ENT consultation. May be due to cholesteatoma or infection with resistant organism (Pseudomonas, S. aureus). In patient with recurrent/chronic draining otitis and evidence of lung infection, consider possibility of immotile cilia syndrome. Only 50% of cases will have situs inversus.

F. Pharyngitis (including tonsillitis and tonsillopharyngitis)

  1. S/sx - May have fever, sore throat, malaise, headache, abd pain, sandpapery rash (scarlet fever). Pharynx will at least be erythematous, $\pm$ tonsillar hypertrophy, $\pm$ exudate, $\pm$ ulcerations, $\pm$ membranous covering, $\pm$ palatal petechiae, cervical adenitis. Antibody rise against Group A beta-hemolytic streptococcus correlates best with enlarged, tender anterior cervical nodes.

  2. Etiology

    a. Bacteria: Group A beta-hemolytic streptococcus - Clinical diagnosis is not reliable to diagnose "strep throat." Patient with strep throat may have fever (often very high), sore throat, headache, + abd pain, vomiting. Pharynx may appear erythematous or exudative; palatal petechiae, tender anterior cervical lymph nodes may be present. Diagnosis of strep throat is based on a positive culture or direct antigen screen and evidence of pharyngitis. Other bacteria: GC - high index of suspicion, positive clinical Hx and PE; diphtheria - membranous pharyngitis, myocarditis, check immunization Hx.

b. Viral:

1) Coxsackie (Herpangina) - usually seen in summer and autumn, ulcers on soft palate, tonsils, pharynx. Also check soles and palms for vesicular lesions: hand-foot-mouth syndrome.

2) Epstein-Barr virus (Infectious Mononucleosis) - may be associated with exudative or membranous pharyngitis, generalized lymphadenopathy, hepatosplenomegaly, rash, malaise, tender posterior cervical nodes, edema of the eyelids, nasal "twang" to voice.

3) Adenovirus - most common cause of nonstrep pharyngitis; may be associated with abd pain, diarrhea, otitis media, rash (duration <3 d).

4) Herpes simplex - both Type I and II may produce pharyngitis ± tonsillar exudate. Ulcerations may appear 1-2 d after onset. If signs of glossitis or gingivostomatitis, probably herpes etiology.

5) Other viruses - ECHO, parainfluenza, influenza, RSV.

c. Other organisms such as mycoplasma.

3. Laboratory Evaluation

a. Throat culture (T/C) is mainstay of diagnosis. NOTE: ~15-18% of children with infectious mono will also have Group A beta-hemolytic streptococcus on T/C.

b. Direct antigen screen may be helpful. Test is very specific (few false-positive results), but false-negative results may be seen in up to 20% of strep infections. Usual strategy - treat if antigen screen positive; if screen is negative, do T/C.

c. cbc + diff + smear (lymphocytosis with atypical lymphs may be seen in ~80% of pt with infectious mononucleosis). Platelets decreased with some viral syndromes. Heterophile monospot (test may be negative before 5 yr or during first wk of illness) or specific serology for EB virus antibody. Consider infectious mono when T/C is neg and severe pharyngitis persists.

4. Treatment
   a. Antibiotics
      1) Important to prevent rheumatic fever if patient has Group A beta-hemolytic streptococcus, but treatment doesn't alter chances of post-strep glomerulonephritis. Antibiotics may shorten duration and severity of symptoms, especially if given early in the course.
         a) 1st choice (100% compliance):
            IM benzathine penicillin 100,000 u/yr to maximum of 1.2 million u. (Comes in containers of 300,000; 600,000; 900,000; 1.2 million. Round dose off to nearest container size).
         b) 2nd choice for patient you know will be compliant:
            Oral penicillin VK 250 mg qid x 10 d
         c) If allergic to penicillin:
            Erythromycin 50 mg/kg/d + qid x 10 d
         d) If patient has all the classic symptoms of strep, you may begin treatment while culture is pending. Generally best to withhold antibiotics until culture results available, unless patient is unlikely to return for follow-up.
   b. Symptomatic treatment
      1) Analgesics, antipyretics.
      2) Throat lozenges, Chloraseptic spray (contains topical anesthetic).

    c. Post-treatment clinical and/or bacteriologic failures
      1) May be due to presence of beta-lactamase-producing organisms in oropharynx
      2) Effective regimens include:
        a) oxacillin,
        b) clindamycin,
        c) dicloxacillin,
        d) benzathine penicillin IM and rifampin,
        e) po penicillin and rifampin.

  5. Miscellaneous
    a. Culture symptomatic family members of pt with strep pharyngitis.
    b. Culture of asymptomatic family members generally not necessary.
    c. 50% of positive throat cultures represent carriers not at risk for rheumatic fever.
    d. Routine post-treatment culture is not indicated. Indications include: family history of rheumatic fever, "ping-ponging" of strep infections in the family, outbreak in closed community, patient being considered for T & A.

G. Sinusitis

  1. Probably present to some degree in all upper respiratory tract infections.
  2. Presentation: purulent rhinorrhea, fetid breath, fever, headache, tenderness over sinuses, cough (during day and worse at night), painless periorbital swelling in morning.
  3. Diagnosis: usually on clinical grounds.
    a. Transillumination - not helpful < 10 yr.
    b. Sinus films - often misleading. If negative, can probably R/O sinusitis. Air-fluid level or mucosal thickening (> 4mm) helpful. Hard to interpret opacification.
    c. Ultrasound or C-T may be helpful in difficult cases.

      d. Sinus aspiration - "Gold standard" - reserve for immunosuppressed patients, patients not responding, or in patients with life-threatening complications.

   4. Bacteriology
Same as OM: <u>S. pneumoniae,</u> non-typable <u>H. influenzae,</u> Group A strep, <u>Branhamella catarrhalis.</u>
N.B. NP and T/C <u>do not</u> correlate with direct sinus aspirate cultures.

   5. Treatment
Same as for OM: amoxicillin, cefaclor, Augmentin, TMP/SMX and Pediazole. In acute infection, a 10-14 day course is usually adequate.

   6. Chronic Sinusitis
     a. Symptoms >30 days.
     b. Anaerobes may be important.
     c. Use same antibiotics, but Rx 3-6 wk.
     d. Role of decongestants and antihistamines is unclear, but may be worth a try.
     e. In teenagers with maxillary sinusitis, think of a dental origin.

H. Upper Respiratory Infection

   1. Supportive measures are the mainstay of therapy.
     a. Rest and fluids.
     b. Humidification (cool mist vaporizer) may soothe inflamed, scratchy nasal and pharyngeal mucosa. Avoid passive smoking and other environmental irritants.
     c. Infants: Buffered saline nose drops $\pm$ bulb syringe. 2 drops in each nostril to loosen secretions, then aspirate with nasal aspirator. Use prior to feeds, bedtime, and prn. NOTE: It is preferable for parents to obtain these drops at pharmacy. Homemade solutions are notorious for being made incorrectly regardless of how simple the recipe, and, therefore, are strongly discouraged.

   d. Analgesics/antipyretics for malaise and fever prn.
2. Antihistamines and/or sympathomimetics
   Efficacy not clearly demonstrated in controlled studies, but often used. Not for use <18 mo age because of hypersensitivity to antihistamine and sympathomimetic effects. Warn parents about drowsiness with antihistamines.
3. Topical decongestants: 0.25% Neo-Synephrine (phenylephrine) nasal drops will decrease mucosal swelling and rhinorrhea. Don't use >3-5 days (tachyphylaxis and rhinitis medicamentosa) or in <6 month old.
4. Cough Medications
   a. Guaifenesin (e.g., plain Robitussin) doesn't work.
   b. Dextromethorphan, a short acting cough suppressant, may help, especially for troublesome nighttime cough.

REFERENCES

Allergic Rhinitis
1. Estelle F, Simons R: Allergic rhinitis: recent advances. *Pediatr Clin N Am* 1988; 35: 1053-1074.
2. Meltzer EO, Zeiger RS, Schatz M, et al: Chronic rhinitis in infants and children: Etiologic, diagnostic, and therapeutic considerations. *Pediatr Clin N Am* 1983; 30: 847-871.
3. Norman P: New developments in treating allergic rhinitis. *Drug Therapy* August 1985.
4. Pearlman DS: Chronic rhinitis in children. *Clin Rev Allergy* 1984; 2: 197-223.
5. Shapiro GG: Understanding allergic rhinitis: Differential diagnosis and management. *Pediatr in Rev* 1986; 7: 212-218.

Epistaxis
1. Barell PA: The management of epistaxis in children. *Otolaryngol Clin North Am* 1977; 10: 91.
2. Culbertson M: Epistaxis in Bluestone CD and Stool SE, Eds. *Pediatric Otolaryngology*, Vol. 1, W.B. Saunders, Philadelphia, 1983.

Foreign Bodies
1. David TJ, Ferguson AP: Management of children who have swallowed button batteries. *Arch Dis Child* 1986; 61: 321-322.
2. Kenna MA, Bluestone CD: Foreign bodies in the air and food passages. *Pediatr in Rev* 1988; 10: 25-31.
3. Litovitz TL: Battery ingestions: Product accessibility and clinical course. *Pediatr* 1985; 75: 469-476.

Hoarseness
1. Passy V: Hoarseness - evaluation and treatment. *Primary Care* 1982; 9: 337-354.

Otitis Media
1. Berman S, Grose K, Zerbe GO: Medical management of chronic middle ear effusion - results of a clinical trial of prednisone combined with sulfamethoxazole and trimethoprim. *Am J Dis Child* 1987; 141: 690-694.
2. Bluestone CD: Otitis media and sinusitis: Management and when to refer to the otolaryngologist. *Pediatr Inf Dis* 1987; 6: 100-106.

3. Cantekin EI, Mandel EM, Bluestone CD, et al: Lack of efficacy of a decongestant-antihistamine combination for otitis media with effusion ("secretory" otitis media) in children. *NEJM* 1983; 308: 297-301.

4. Chang MG, Rodriguez WJ, Mohla: <u>Chlamydia trachomatis</u> in otitis media in children. *Pediatr Inf Dis* 1982; 1: 95-97.

5. Klein BS, Dollette FR, Yolken RH: The role of respiratory syncytial virus and other viral pathogens in acute otitis media. *J Pediatr* 1982; 101: 16-20.

6. Kovatch AL, Wald ER, Michaels RH: Beta-lactamase-producing Branhamella catarrhalis causing otitis media in children.J Pediatr 1983; 102: 261-265.

7. Liston TE, Foshee WS, Pierson MWD: Sulfisoxazole chemoprophylaxis and recurrent otitis media. *Pediatr* 1983; 71: 524-530.

8. Mandel EM, Rockette HE, Bluestone CD, et al: Efficacy of amoxicillin with and without decongestant - antihistamine for otitis media with effusion in children - results of a double-blind, randomized trial. *NEJM* 1987; 316: 432-437.

9. Nelson JD: Changing trends in the microbiology and management of acute otitis media and sinusitis. *Pediatr Inf Dis* 1986; 5: 749-753.

10. Perrin JM, et al: Sulfisoxazole as chemoprophylaxis for recurrent otitis media. *NEJM* 1974; 291: 664-667.

11. Riding KH, Bluestone CD, Michaels RJ, et al: Microbiology of recurrent and chronic otitis media with effusion. *J Pediatr* 1978; 93: 739-743.

12. Schwartz RH, Puglese J, Schwartz DM: Use of a short course of prednisone for treating middle ear effusion: A double-blind crossover study. 1980; 89: 296-300.

13. Shurin PA, et al: Bacterial etiology of otitis media in first 6 weeks of life. *J Pediatr* 1978; 92: 893.

14. Sunberg L: Antibiotic treatment of secretory otitis media. *Acta Otolaryngol* [Suppl] (Stockholm) 1984; 407: 26-29.

15. Teele DW, Teele J: Detection of middle ear effusion by acoustic reflectometry. *J Pediatr* 1984; 104: 832.

16. Tetzlaff, Ashworth C, Nelson JO: Otitis media in children under 12 weeks of age. *Pediatr* 1977; 59: 827.

Pharyngitis
1. Chaudhary S, Bilinsky SA, Hennessy JL, et al: Penicillin V and rifampin for the treatment of Group A streptococcal pharyngitis: a randomized trial of 10 days of penicillin vs 10 days penicillin with rifampin during the final 4 days of therapy. *J Pediatr* 1985; 106: 481.
2. Grose C: The many faces of infectious mononucleosis: The spectrum of Epstein-Barr virus infection in children. *Pediatr in Rev* 1984; 7: 35-44.
3. Kaplan EG, Gastanaduy AS, Howe BB: The rule of the carrier in treatment failure after antibiotic therapy for Group A streptococci in the upper respiratory tract. *J Lab Clin Med* 1981; 98: 326.
4. Kaplan EL: The rapid identification of Group A beta-hemolytic streptococci in the upper respiratory tract. *Pediatr Clin N Am* 1988; 35: 535-542.
5. McCracken GH: Diagnosis and management of children with streptococcal pharyngitis. *Ped Inf Dis* 1987; 5: 754.
6. Randolph MF, Gerber MA, DeMeo KK, et al: Effect of antibiotic therapy on the clinical course of streptococcal pharyngitis. *J Pediatr* 1985; 106: 870.
7. Sumaya CU, Ench Y: Epstein-Barr virus infectious mononucleosis in children: Clinical and general laboratory findings. *Pediatr* 1985; 75: 1003-1010.

Sinusitis
1. Brook I: Bacteriologic features of chronic sinusitis in children. *JAMA* 1981; 246: 967-970.
2. Wald ER: Acute and chronic sinusitis: Diagnosis and management. *Pediatr in Rev* 1984; 7: 150-157.
3. Wald ER, Milmoe GH, Bowen A, et al: Acute maxillary sinusitis in children. *NEJM* 1981; 304: 749-754.

17

PULMONARY

A. Apnea

1. Apnea is the cessation of respiratory airflow. May be due to:
   a. Absence of respiratory effort (central)
   b. Obstruction of the airway (obstructive)
   c. Combination of both (mixed)

   Occasional respiratory pauses of 15 seconds or less may be a normal finding at any age. If apnea lasts >20 seconds or is accompanied by bradycardia, pallor, hypotonia, or cyanosis it is termed pathological apnea.

   ALTE - (apparent life-threatening episode; formerly called "near miss sudden infant death syndrome" SIDS). Refers to an episode of apnea that is frightening to the observer and that requires vigorous stimulation or resuscitative efforts. (Not all apnea leads to ALTEs and not all ALTEs involve apnea). No evidence that apnea alone increases the risk for SIDS, but infants with ALTEs are at increased risk for sudden death.

2. Etiology of ALTEs

Acute Infection (sepsis, pneumonia, meningitis)

RSV bronchiolitis

GE reflux with aspiration

Dysfunctional swallowing with aspiration

Seizures

Disorders of respiratory control (central)

Anemia

Metabolic disorder

Respiratory disease (BPD)

Cardiac disease

Poisoning

CNS tumors

Upper airway obstruction

3. Approach to child with ALTE

Unless there is evidence to suggest otherwise, the parents' and/or caretakers' observations must be considered valid and accurate. Parental anxiety should not be minimized.

First need to R/O treatable causes of such events.

a. Careful history - focus on circumstances of event; perinatal history; family history. (Awake apnea suggests seizures or reflux/aspiration.)

b. Physical exam - focus on upper airway, cardiac, pulmonary, and neurologic exam; observe feeding and sleeping pattern.

c. Lab studies - minimum w/u involves:

CBC and diff

Blood glucose/electrolytes/bicarbonate

Based on initial evaluation, additional w/u may include:

Barium swallow

Chest x-ray

Electrocardiogram

Electroencephalogram

Esophageal pH probe

Sleep study

Upper airway evaluation

All infants with an ALTE should be admitted for at least 48 h for evaluation, monitoring, and parental CPR instruction.

Once an infant has presented with an ALTE, the likelihood is that it will happen again.

N.B. A negative exam and lab w/u does not indicate that a significant event did not occur or that it will not happen again. If no etiology is found, the infant will still require long-term monitoring.

Recovery from an apnea episode with only minimal intervention suggests that what was witnessed was a normal physiologic event. If exam and minimal lab w/u (see above) are normal, such infants may be discharged home without an extensive w/u.

1) Need to be supportive of family, answer questions patiently, and ensure adequate F/U.

2) Parents should be included in the decision-making process.

4. Munchausen by proxy

Be suspicious if there is a history of 2 or more episodes of apnea requiring resuscitation that began only in the presence of the parent but were then witnessed by other persons subsequently called for assistance. Strong evidence that these cases may be related to child abuse (Munchausen by proxy).

Clues include:

a. History of multiple resuscitations (especially in hospital setting)

b. No recognized cardiorespiratory abnormalities between episodes

c. Episodes began only in the parent's presence

d. Resuscitation witnessed by others

e. Siblings with similar episodes or death

f. One of the parents (usually the mother) is medically sophisticated and shows exemplary behavior in the medical setting.

B. Asthma

1. Hx - If pt is in acute distress, take brief, pertinent history. (Calm child down.) When did wheezing begin? Precipitating events (e.g., URI, allergen, irritants, exercise, change in weather, etc.?) Is child a known asthmatic or is this a "first-time" wheezer? Any associated illness? Family history of atopy (asthma, hay fever, eczema). Medications? Last dose? Course of previous episodes? Previous hospitalizations for asthma? What type of ER or inpatient regimen has usually reversed patient's acute attack?

   If this is first wheezing event, consider in differential diagnosis possibility of foreign body aspiration, CHF, bronchiolitis, CF - especially if wheezing is atypical, not responding to therapy, and negative family hx for atopy. Has child had chronic cough?(Some asthmatics will present this way without overt wheezing.)

2. PE - Vital Signs (All of them)

   Assess degree of severity: supraclavicular retractions correlate well with degree of obstruction; cyanotic?; tightness (some patients may be so tight, i.e., poor air movement, that no wheezing is heard); measure peak flow (if >6 yr old); pulsus paradoxus (significant bronchospasm produces pulsus >15 mm Hg). Evaluate state of hydration and mental status.

3. Lab - In patient who has been on theophylline preparation, obtain serum theophylline level.

   In cooperative child, peak flow rate may be helpful. If peak flow is <30% predicted or does not increase to 40% predicted after Rx, often predicts need for admission.

   In patient with evidence of severe obstruction or change in mental status, ABGs should be obtained. PO_2 <50 mmHg or PCO_2 >40 mmHg indicates respiratory failure. A normal or slightly elevated

PCO_2 in a hyperventilating child may be a sign of impending respiratory failure.

4. Chest X-ray - Not generally helpful and not indicated as a routine procedure. X-ray findings do not correlate with severity of attack. X-rays may be indicated for:
   a. Initial episode of wheezing
   b. Temperature >38.5
   c. Localized or persistent rales - especially in child over 2 yr
   d. Patient who appears especially ill or does not respond to Rx as expected.

5. ER Treatment - Maintain calm environment. Hydrate if patient is dry (usually po). If patient is in distress, administer humidified O_2 (100%) by face mask. Keep flow sheet of Rx and response - check vital signs and physical findings at frequent intervals.

MEDICATIONS

Epinephrine	Comes as 1: 1000 dilution of aqueous epinephrine	0.01 cc/kg SQ. Maximum single dose 0.3 cc.	
Susphrine	1: 200 dilution of long-acting microcrystalline epinephrine	0.005 cc/kg SQ. Maximum dose 0.15 cc.	Shake vial well to avoid settling suspension.
Isoetharine (Bronkosol)	1% for inhalation	Dilute 1: 4 with saline. Maximum dose - 5 minutes inhalation. Use flow rate of 4-6 1/min. of O_2.	Short-acting-glh. May repeat in 1/2 hour.
Aminophylline	IV	Bolus of 6 mg/kg Followed by constant infusion of 1 mg/kg/hr	Dilute in 25-50 cc of saline and give bolus over 20 minutes.
Hydrocortisone	IV	7 mg/kg stat dose. Followed by 5-7 mg/kg/24 hr	

Traditional therapy consists of series of SQ epinephrine injections, but <u>no difference</u> between SQ epinephrine and inhalations of ß2 agonists (bronkosol, metaproterenol, terbutaline). <u>NEBULIZATION THERAPY SHOULD BE TREATMENT OF CHOICE.</u>
In patient who is uncooperative with nebulization, substitute SQ aqueous epinephrine - 0.01 cc/kg (maximum dose 0.3 cc). This dose may be repeated x 2. If patient clears, give susphrine 0.005 cc/kg SQ (maximum dose 0.15cc) and send home. If patient does not clear, go to IV aminophylline.

NEUBULIZATION PROTOCOL

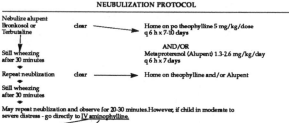

Nebulize alupent Bronkosol or Terbutaline — clear → Home on po theophylline 5 mg/kg/dose q 6 h x 7-10 days

AND/OR
Metaproterenol (Alupent) 1.3-2.6 mg/kg/day q 6 h x 7 days

Still wheezing after 30 minutes

Repeat neublization — clear → Home on theophylline and/or Alupent

Still wheezing after 30 minutes

May repeat neublization and observe for 20-30 minutes. However, if child in moderate to severe distress - go directly to IV aminophylline.

clear ←
persistent wheezing

home on po theophylline and/or Alupent and/or short course po Prednisone

ADMIT

Dose depends on previous theophylline Rx - always get pre-bolus serum level.
1 mg/kg of aminophylline will raise serum concentration 2 micrograms/ml. Usual bolus is 6 mg/kg followed by a constant IV infusion of 1 mg/kg/hr. Be sure to get post-bolus level. If level is low, re-bolus. If wheezing persists, Alupent or Bronkosol neublization can be repeated q 1-2 h. If patient is not responding or PO2 <60 in room air, add IV hydrocortisone. Watch for theophylline side effects - mainly vomiting.

In general, decision to send home or admit should be made within 4 hours of arrival in ER, unless a 24-hour holding unit is available.

EPINEPHRINE PROTOCOL

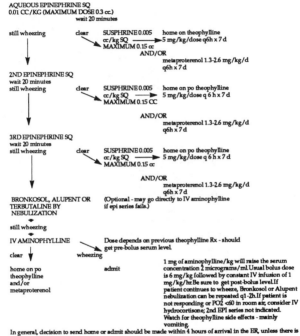

AQUEOUS EPINEPHRINE SQ
0.01 CC/KG (MAXIMUM DOSE 0.3 cc.)
　　　　　　　wait 20 minutes

still wheezing　　　　　clear　　SUSPHRINE 0.005　　home on theophylline
　　　　　　　　　　　　　　　　cc/kg SQ ──────► 5 mg/kg/dose q6h x 7 d
　　　　　　　　　　　　　　　　MAXIMUM 0.15 cc

　　　　　　　　　　　　　　　　　　　　AND/OR

　　　　　　　　　　　　　　　　　　　　metaproterenol 1.3-2.6 mg/kg/d
　　　　　　　　　　　　　　　　　　　　q6h x 7 d

2ND EPINEPHRINE SQ
wait 20 minutes
still wheezing　　　　　clear　　SUSPHRINE 0.005　　home on po theophylline
　　　　　　　　　　　　　　　　cc/kg SQ ────── 5 mg/kg/dose q 6 h x 7 d
　　　　　　　　　　　　　　　　MAXIMUM 0.15 CC

　　　　　　　　　　　　　　　　　　　　AND/OR

　　　　　　　　　　　　　　　　　　　　metaproterenol 1.3-2.6 mg/kg/d
　　　　　　　　　　　　　　　　　　　　q6h x 7 d

3RD EPINEPHRINE SQ
wait 20 minutes
still wheezing　　　　　clear　　SUSPHRINE 0.005　　home on po theophylline
　　　　　　　　　　　　　　　　cc/kg SQ ────── 5 mg/kg/dose q 6 h x 7 d
　　　　　　　　　　　　　　　　MAXIMUM 0.15 cc

　　　　　　　　　　　　　　　　　　　　AND/OR

　　　　　　　　　　　　　　　　　　　　metaproterenol 1.3-2.6 mg/kg/d
　　　　　　　　　　　　　　　　　　　　q6h x 7 d

BRONKOSOL, ALUPENT OR　　(Optional - may go directly to IV aminophylline
TERBUTALINE BY　　　　　　if epi series fails.)
NEBULIZATION

still wheezing

IV AMINOPHYLLINE　　　　Dose depends on previous theophylline Rx - should
　　　　　　　　　　　　　get pre-bolus serum level.

clear　　　　wheezing

home on po　　　admit　　　1 mg of aminophylline/kg will raise the serum
theophylline　　　　　　　concentration 2 micrograms/ml. Usual bolus dose
and/or　　　　　　　　　is 6 mg/kg followed by constant IV infusion of 1
metaproterenol　　　　　mg/kg/hr. Be sure to get post-bolus level. If
　　　　　　　　　　　　patient continues to wheeze, Bronkosol or Alupent
　　　　　　　　　　　　nebulization can be repeated q1-2h. If patient is
　　　　　　　　　　　　not responding or PO2 <60 in room air, consider IV
　　　　　　　　　　　　hydrocortisone; 2nd EPI series not indicated.
　　　　　　　　　　　　Watch for theophylline side effects - mainly
　　　　　　　　　　　　vomiting.

In general, decision to send home or admit should be made within 4 hours of arrival in the ER, unless there is
a 24 hour holding unit.
Alternative to the epinephrine protocol is to administer Bronkosol, Alupent, or terbutaline by nebulization:
may repeat in 1/2 hour. If not clear, go to IV aminophylline. Nebulization protocol should be used in cooperative patients.

6. Miscellaneous
   a. Theophylline preparations are the mainstay of therapy: dozens of preparations available: consult *Harriet Lane Handbook* for names and dosages. Serum levels should be checked.
   b. Sustained-release preparations preferable for chronic use. Do not prescribe long-acting preparations for PRN use.
   c. Terbutaline is useful β_2 adrenergic agonist.2.5 mg/dose po tid (not approved for <12 yr). Useful agent for patients allergic to metabisulfite.
   d. Cromolyn. For prophylaxis only. 20 mg by nebulization q6-8 h. Most effective with exercise-induced asthma.
   e. Steroids
      1) Prednisone 1-1.5 mg/kg/d. For short period (7-10 d). Useful in patient with frequent visits at short intervals. Give entire daily dose in AM - full dose x 3-5 d - taper quickly.
      2) Beclomethasone inhaler 1-2 puffs q6-8h. May allow tapering of oral steroids in steroid-dependent patient.

C. Bronchiolitis

Acute onset of respiratory distress with cough, tachypnea, retractions, wheezing, rales, irritability, nasal discharge. Apnea may occur in up to 20% of cases.
1. History - ? associated or underlying illness of child. Look for Hx of atopy in patient and/or family.
2. PE - Assess degree of respiratory distress. Tachypnea? Flaring? Retractions? Decreased air entry, lethargy, and cyanosis are bad signs. Good correlation between severity of retractions and degree of hypoxemia.
3. Lab - Not usually helpful. ABGs indicated in patient with severe distress. CXR indicated in patients with moderate to severe distress.
4. Etiology - Usually viral; RSV infection usual cause; parainfluenza; occasionally <u>Mycoplasma.</u>

5. Treatment - Hard to differentiate from first episode of asthma.
    a. In patients <15 months, bronchodilators may not be effective. However, epinephrine 0.01 cc/kg or nebulization with alupent may be tried; if helpful, follow with po alupent.
    b. Some evidence that combination of oral steroid and inhaled B_2 agent may be effective.
    c. Most patients can be managed at home.
    d. Indications for admission include: dehydration, secondary bacterial infection, marked respiratory distress (PO_2 <70).
    e. In hospitalized patients, treatment consists of O_2, hydration, and good nursing care.
    f. Need to consider course of nebulized ribavirin in high risk patients, i.e., underyling congenital heart disease, BPD, etc.

D. Croup

Acute onset of inspiratory stridor, "barky" cough, hoarseness, retractions - often follows URI.
1. Etiology
    a. Viral (most common) - parainfluenza, RSV, adenovirus.
    b. Spasmodic (? allergic).
    c. Bacterial - staphylococcal, <u>H. influenzae.</u>
    d. If recurrent, R/O foreign body or congenital subglottic stenosis.
2. PE - Assess degree of distress, hydration, general activity, hypotonia, air entry, retractions, lethargy, tachycardia out of proportion to fever, cyanosis.
3. Lab - Not usually helpful. Radiograph of upper airway not indicated in all cases.
4. Management - Calm child (and family) - avoid painful procedures.
    a. Most important is humidification with cool mist.
    b. Use of steroids is controversial; but generally indicated (dexamethasone 0.6 mg/kg IM x 1).

c. Racemic epinephrine (2%) - 0.5 cc added to 3 cc water and delivered by nebulization may give transient relief (1-2 h) but often followed by rebound; best reserved for patients being Rx in hospital (not ER).

d. Do not use sedation.

e. Indications for admission include dehydration and/or evidence of respiratory compromise i.e., cyanosis, fatigue, hypotonia, PCO_2 >45, PO_2 <70.

E. **Epiglottitis: A true pediatric emergency! The initial goal is to establish and maintain a good airway. A physician must accompany the patient at all times.**

1. Classic presentation
   a. Fulminant course in previously well child.
   b. Stridor, respiratory distress (within hours of onset); high fever; typical posturing is a child preferring to sit (don't make patient lie down!), head forward, open mouth, drooling, anxious appearance, dysphagia (will refuse to drink).
   c. Age onset: range 7 mo - 10 yr (avg. 3 yr)
   d. Differentiate from <u>croup,</u> which does <u>not</u> have such a rapid evolution; croup also has more coughing and hoarseness; stridor may be similar to epiglottitis. Although croup may be severe, usually child is not in the degree of distress that is seen in epiglottitis.

2. Initial Mangement: Minimize disturbance, keep child calm, and avoid attempts to visualize pharynx or epiglottis.
   a. If child has classic presentation, ENT and/or anesthesiology should be notified.
   b. If presentation is not straightforward and child is not in severe distress, obtain stat x-ray <u>(lateral view)</u> of the neck with patient <u>erect</u> (not supine).

   If lateral view confirms epiglottitis, call ENT and/or anesthesiology.

   c. <u>All</u> patients with documented epiglottitis need an artificial airway regardless of the degree of distress at the time of evaluation - they can decompensate quickly. The airway should be placed in the OR.

   d. If a patient is clinically <u>suspected</u> of having epiglottitis, the following protocol is followed:

      1) EXAMINATION OF THE PHARYNX IS PRO-HIBITED ONCE EPIGLOTTITIS IS SUSPECT-ED. Minimize disturbance; keep the patient upright; unobtrusively administer facial O_2 (blow-by). <u>Do not</u> draw blood or place intravenous lines; do not give po fluids.

      2) The patient should never be left without a physician in attendance. Parents are often helpful in relieving the child's anxiety. <u>Do not crowd</u> the child.

      3) When the child is transported for any reason, he/she should be accompanied by pediatrician, ENT, anesthesiologist. Airway equipment should be on hand. (Ambu bag, laryngoscope, and ET tube, and 14 gauge angiocath for emergency tracheotomy). The patient should be transported in the <u>upright</u> position, with <u>minimum disturbance</u>, and with oxygen unobtrusively administered.

Clinical Guidelines: Epiglottitis vs Croup (Laryngotracheobronchitis)		
	Epiglottitis	Croup
AGE	May affect all ages	Younger children
	Peak: 3-5 yr	3 mo - 3 yr
ETIOLOGY	Bacterial (H. influenzae)	Viral (parainfluenza)
SITE OF INFLAMMATION	Supraglottic	Subglottic
ONSET OF RESP SX	Usually rapid (30 min-6h)	Slow (1-4 d)
SYMPTOMS: Appearance	Anxious, ill, toxic	Frequently non-toxic
Position	Upright, forward	Variable
Temperature	Usually high (>39°C)	Normal to high
Resp distress	Usually present	Variable
Retractions	Usually late finding	Progressive
Voice/Cough	Muffled/often absent	Hoarse/"seal bark"
Mouth	Open jaw, forward, may drool	Closed, nasal flaring

Frequency of Symptoms in Combined Series of Epiglottitis Patients (N=319)			
Fever:	85%	Dysphagia:	40%
Respiratory distress:	80%	Drooling:	37%
Retractions:	59%	Cyanosis:	33%
Stridor:	54%	Cough:	25%
Sore throat:	46%	Hoarseness:	23%

F Foreign Body Aspiration

1. Presentation
   a. Signs and symptoms include wheezing, cough, and evidence of chest infection. May present with hemoptysis. A choking episode is observed in only 50-80% of cases often leading to a delay in diagnosis.
   b. Usual age is 6 mo to 3 yr.
   c. Most common objects are peanuts.
   d. Always suspect a FB if a pneumonia does not resolve completely or recurs after antibiotic is stopped.
2. Diagnosis
   a. History is crucial but often not obtained or appreciated.
   b. Diagnostic triad includes coughing, localized wheezing, and locally diminished or absent breath sounds.
   c. CXR may show air trapping, atelectasis, or pneumonia. A radio-opaque object is seen in ~ 15% of cases.

N.B. Left-sided aspiration is almost as common as right-sided, and the CXR is entirely negative in 20% of cases.

    d. Inspiratory and expiratory films and fluoroscopy may be helpful. However, if suspicious of FB and initial evaluation is negative, refer for bronchoscopy.

3. Management

    a. Rigid bronchoscopy is procedure of choice.

    b. Because of the possibility of airway obstruction, chest physiotherapy should not be carried out prior to endoscopy.

    N.B. There may be more than one foreign body. Endoscopist needs to look on both sides.

4. Button Battery Ingestions

New hazard of the electronic age. May cause rapid tissue destruction either by leakage of alkaline contents or by tissue electrolysis caused by low-voltage direct current. If there is history of a battery ingestion, the first step is to x-ray chest and abdomen to localize the cell; remember, more than one cell may have been ingested.

    a. If a battery is lodged in the esophagus, immediate removal is indicated. Endoscopy is the procedure of choice; use of a magnet may be helpful.

    b. Virtually all batteries that reach the stomach will be passed without complication.

        1) An X-ray should be obtained daily to document passage.

        2) If the cell remains fixed to the gastric mucosa for a prolonged period, it will need to be removed, probably by endoscopy, but this has been accomplished by attaching a magnet to an N/G tube.

        3) An antacid should be given to prevent corrosion.

        4) No evidence that metoclopramide or an H_2 blocker are helpful.

    c. All cells that pass the pylorus will pass through the gut without problem.

      1) Laxatives and enemas may speed process (controversial).

      2) Parents should exam stools for the cell.

      3) An X-ray should be obtained every 4 d until the cell is recovered.

G. Hemoptysis

    1. Although a rare event, can be life threatening. May be confused with hematemesis.

	Hemoptysis	Hematemesis
color	bright red	dark red
pH	alkaline	acid
appearance	frothy	+/- food particles
symptoms	cough	nausea, retching

N.B. Always think of a pulmonary source of bleeding in children with unexplained hematemesis.

    2. Differential Diagnosis

      a. In children, most likely causes are infection and aspirated foreign bodies.

      b. In infants and young children, need to think of tumors, A-V malformations, cysts, and hemosiderosis (hemoptysis, infiltrates, iron deficiency anemia).

    3. Evaluation

      a. Careful history.

      b. Always start exam at the top - nasopharynx is often source of bleeding.

      c. Check skin for hemangiomata, telangiectases, signs of trauma.

      d. CXR is test with highest yield. However, a normal CXR does not R/O a pulmonary source of bleeding.

      Except in cases of blood-tinged sputum or mild bleeding, patient with hemoptysis should be admitted. If initial evaluation is negative, bronchoscopy will be necessary.

H. Pneumonia

1. Hx - may be <u>acute</u> or <u>subacute</u> onset, fever $\pm$ chills, cough, difficult or rapid breathing, $\pm$ pain on inspiration, malaise. Ask about exposure to TB, previous pneumonia.

2. PE - All vital signs.
   a. Tachypnea - very sensitive clinical sign, but may be associated with other disorders (e.g., DKA, salicylate poisoning, foreign body, bronchiolitis, asthma).
   b. Rales are frequently present, but may be absent depending upon type of pneumonic process.
   c. Sputum production rare in very young children (i.e., <6 yr).
   d. Shallow breathing or splinting secondary to pleuritic pain.
   e. Localized findings of decreased breath sounds, dullness to percussion.
   f. Look for other sites of infection (OM, conjunctivitis, etc.)

3. Lab
   a. CXR: Infiltrate may not be present early in illness. Infiltrates may be lobar, segmental, nodular, miliary, interstitial, perihilar, etc. Other significant findings include pleural effusion, pneumatoceles (can be seen with many bacteria - not just <u>S. aureus</u>), cavitations. In most cases the CXR cannot differentiate among bacterial, viral, mycoplasma and chalmydia pneumonias. CXR is not indicated in all patients with suspected pneumonia - most are diagnosed clinically.
   b. TB skin test: Indicated in patients with chronic or complicated pneumonia, those with a positive family history, and in other high risk groups (i.e., immigrants from Southeast Asia).

c. CBC: WBC may be higher in bacterial vs. viral pneumonias, but there is a great deal of overlap and results will usually not alter Rx. Moderate eosinophilia may be present in chlamydia, parasitic, allergic, or hypersensitivity pneumonias.

d. Blood culture: Not done routinely; will be positive in only 5-10% of patients with presumed bacterial pneumonia. Consider clinical setting, i.e., age, fever, WBC count, toxic appearance.

e. Cold Agglutinins: Used as a screening test for <u>M. pneumoniae,</u> but does not discriminate well between mycoplasma and viral infections.

f. CIE: Serum or urine CIE or slide agglutination tests for pneumococcal and <u>H. influenzae</u> antigen can help establish a bacterial etiology but is not practical in most outpatient settings.

g. <u>Chlamydia</u> studies: Conjunctival scraping or NP swab may be Giemsa stained or cultured (special media required) for <u>Chlamydia</u>. Fluorescent antibody microscopy of NP secretions correlates well with culture results.

h. Cultures: NP culture is worthless. Sputum culture and Gram stain may be helpful if a good sputum (not saliva) specimen is obtained.

Tracheal aspirate is rarely used in children. Probably better than sputum but still may be contaminated with upper respiratory secretions.

Lung puncture occasionally reveals organism but not routinely used.

Pleural effusions should be tapped and sent for culture, AFB and Gram stain, chemistries, and cytology.

Lung biopsy is indicated in highly selected, complicated cases.

i. C-reactive protein: In general, elevation of CRP is indicative of bacterial infection, but there is considerable overlap.

4. Etiology

Conclusive evidence is difficult to obtain in children. Etiology may be suspected on basis of clinical presentation and community outbreaks. Among pediatric outpatients presenting with pneumonia, approximately 10-20% will be due to a bacterial agent. Most will be due to viral agents - influenza, parainfluenza, adenovirus, and RSV (especially in infants). In about 10% of children there will be coexistent viral and bacterial infection. In older children (>8 yr) and adolescents, <u>M. pneumoniae</u> is a common etiologic agent.

a. Bacterial: Acute onset of symptoms with significant fever and lobar consolidation suggests bacterial pneumonia. Most common organisms (based on lung punctures and blood cultures) are <u>S. pneumoniae</u> and <u>H. influenzae</u>. <u>S. aureus</u> should be considered in young or debilitated infants, especially if effusions or pneumatoceles are present. Streptococcal pneumonia may be associated with scarlatiniform rash; blood culture and pleural fluid cultures may be positive, but T/C is often negative.

b. Viral: Viral etiologies include adenovirus, influenza, parainfluenza and RSV. In older children, there is usually a non-productive cough and systemic symptoms such as myalgias, headaches, coryza, fatigue, and general malaise.In infants, wheezing is often a prominent feature.

c. <u>Chlamydia:</u> <u>C. trachomatis</u> may be responsible for 15-30% of afebrile pneumonias in early infancy. The typical patient is afebrile with a staccato cough, peripheral eosinophilia, and diffuse interstitial infiltrates. Half of the patients will have conjunctivitis.

d. Mycoplasma: Common in school age children and young adults. Characterized by gradual onset, low grade or absent fever, interstitial

infiltrates, and greater severity of symptoms.
e. Fungal, protozoal, and TB infections must be considered in chronic pneumonia.

In general, viral and bacterial etiologies cannot be reliably distinguished on the basis of clinical picture, laboratory results, or radiographic findings. In addition to investigating etiology, consider underlying disease process predisposing patient to chronic, persistent, or recurrent pneumonias, e.g., immune compromise (congenital, iatrogenic), CF, TEF, GER, foreign body, lobar emphysema, bronchogenic cyst. Also, remember that not all infiltrates are infectious (e.g., metastases, lymphoma).

5. Treatment
    a. Whom to admit
       Infants less than 2 mo should be hospitalized and treated with antibiotics after appropriate sepsis evaluation. Antibiotic choice varies with clinical presentation of patient and physician's differential dx. Would want to consider coverage for strep, <u>H. influenzae,</u> <u>Pneumococcus,</u> staph, <u>E. coli,</u> and <u>Chlamydia.</u> Certainly any patient who appears very ill, has significant respiratory compromise, or is toxic should be admitted. Also, those with progression of pneumonia during outpatient Rx, presence of other complicating factors, or unreliable parents should be admitted.
    b. For most children, outpatient therapy is appropriate. Prudent clinical practice is to treat pneumonia of mild-to-moderate severity as if it is bacterial and not to carry out extensive laboratory evaluation. For young children, initial therapy with amoxicillin plus clavulanate potassium (Augmentin) or cefaclor (Ceclor) - 30-40 mg/kg/d ÷ tid x 10d is appropriate. An alternate approach is to start with ampicillin and switch to Augmentin or cefaclor if there is no improvement after 48 hr. In the event of peni-

cillin allergy, in children >8 yr and in young infants with suspected Chlamydia infection, treatment with erythromycin (50 mg/kg/d) alone or in combination with sulfisoxazole (150 mg/kg/d) qid x 10d is appropriate initial therapy.

c. General supportive care: Rest, antipyretics if necessary. Cough suppressant not recommended for pneumonia. Expectorants don't work. Hydration.

d. Follow-up in 1-2 d.
   1) If improved, see again at completion of therapy. Uncomplicated bacterial pneumonia should improve in 24-48 hr.
   2) Consider inadequate therapy, incorrect diagnosis, or noncompliance if no improvement or progression of process.
   3) Follow-up CXR: Usually not necessary unless patient has persistent symptoms, recurrent pneumonia, or FTT. In one study, 20% of children had residual infiltrates 3-4 wk after acute pneumonia, though clinically better; 100% had cleared within 3 mo.
   4) Remember to put TB skin test on patient if one has not recently been placed.

REFERENCES

Apnea
1. Bruhn FW, et al: Apnea associated with respiratory syncytial virus infection in young infants. *J Pediatr* 1977; 90: 382.
2. Herbst JJ, et al: Gastroesophageal reflux in the "near miss" sudden infant death syndrome. *J Pediatr* 1978; 92: 73.
3. NIH consensus development conference on infantile apnea and home monitoring. *Pediatr* 1987; 79: 292.
4. Rosen CL, Frust JD, Bricker T, et al: Two siblings with recurrent cardiopulmonary arrest: Munchausen by proxy or child abuse? *Pediatr* 1983; 71: 715.

Asthma
1. Becker AB, et al: Inhaled salbutamol (albuterol) vs. injected epinephrine in the treatment of acute asthma in children. *J Pediatr* 1983; 102: 465-469.
2. Ben-Zvi Z, Lam C, Hoffman J, et al: An evaluation of the initial treatment of acute asthma. *Pediatr* 1982; 70: 348-353.
3. Ellis EF: Asthma: Current therapeutic approach. *Pediatr Clin N Am* 1988; 35: 1041-1052.
4. Galant SP, Groncy CE, Shaw KC: The value of pulsus paradoxus in assessing the child with status asthmaticus. *Pediatr* 1978; 61: 46-51.
5. Kattan M, Gurwitz D, Levison H: Corticosteroids in status asthmaticus. *J Pediatr* 1980; 96: 596-599.
6. Kelly HW: New beta-2-agonist aerosols. *Clin Pharm* 1985; 4: 393.
7. Leffert F: The management of acute asthma. *J Pediatr* 1980; 96: 1-12.
8. Murphy SA, Kelly HW: Cromolyn sodium: A review of mechanisms and clinical use in asthma. *Drug Intell Clin Pharm* 1987; 21: 22-35.
9. Zwerdling RG: Status asthmaticus. *Pediatr Ann* 1986; 15: 105-109.

Bronchiolitis
1. Fireman P: The wheezing infant. *Pediatr in Rev* 1986; 6: 247-255.
2. Hall CB, McBride JT, Walsh EE, et al: Aerosolized ribavirin treatment of infants with respiratory syncytial viral infection. *NEJM* 1983; 308: 1443-1447.

3. Outwater KM, Crome RK: Management of respiratory failure in infants with acute viral bronchiolitis. *Am J Dis Child* 1984; 138: 1071-1075.
4. Silverman M: Bronchodilators for wheezing infants? *Arch Dis Child* 1984; 59: 84-87.
5. Tala, Bavilski C, Yohai, et al: Dexamethasone and salbutamol in the treatment of acute wheezing in infants. *Pediatr* 1983; 7: 13-18.
6. Wohl ME: Bronchiolitis. *Pediatr Ann* 1986; 15: 307-313.
7. Wohl ME, Chernick V: State of the art: Bronchioloitis. *Am Rev Resp Dis* 1978; 118: 759.

Croup and Epiglottitis

1. Battaglia JD: Severe croup: The child with fever and upper airway obstruction. *Pediatr in Rev* 1986; 7: 227-233.
2. Davis HW, Gartner JC, Galvis AG, et al: Acute upper airway obstruction: Croup and epiglottitis. *Pediatr Clin N Am* 1981; 28: 859-880.
3. Gardner HG, Powell KR, Roden VJ: The evaluation of racemic epinephrine in the treatment of infectious croup. *Pediatr* 1973; 52: 52.
4. Hen J Jr: Current management of upper airway obstruction. *Pediatr Annals* 1986; 15: 274-294.
5. Newth CJL, Levison H: Croup and epiglottitis. *J Resp Dis* 1981; 2: 22.
6. Rapkin R: The diagnosis of epiglottitis.*J Pediatr* 1972; 80: 96.
7. Tunnessen WW Jr, Feinstein AR: The steroid-croup controversy: An analytic review of methodologic problems. *J Pediatr* 1980; 96: 751.

Foreign body aspiration

1. Blazer S, Haven Y, Friedman A: Foreign body in the airway. *Am J Dis Child* 1980; 134: 68.
2. Gay BB, Atkinson GO, Vanderzalm T, et al: Subglottic foreign bodies in pediatric patients. *Am J Dis Child* 1986; 140;165-168.
3. Laks Y, Barzilay A: Foreign body aspiration in childhood. *Pediatr Emerg Care* 1988; 4: 102-106.

Hemoptysis

1. Beckerman RC, Taussig LM, Pinnas JL: Familial idiopathic pulmonary hemosiderosis. *Am J Dis Child* 1979; 133: 609-611.

2. Metz SJ, Rosenstein BJ: Uncovering the cause of hemoptysis in children. *J Resp Dis* 1984; 5: 43-51.

3. Pyman C: Inhaled foreign bodies in childhood. *Med J Australia* 1971; 1: 62-68.

4. Tom LWC, Weisman RA, Handler SD: Hemoptysis in children. *Ann Otolaryn* 1980; 89: 419-424.

Pneumonia

1. Broughton RA: Infections due to mycoplasma pneumoniae in childhood. *Pediatr Inf Dis* 1986; 5: 71-85.

2. Cherian T, et al: Simple clinical signs of acute lower respiratory tract infection. *Lancet* 1988; 2: 125.

3. Cohen GJ: Management of infections of the lower respiratory tract in children. *Pediatr Inf Dis* 1987; 6: 317-323.

4. Denny FW: Acute respiratory infections in children: Etiology and epidemiology. *Pediatr in Rev* 1987; 9;135-146.

5. Gooch M III: Bronchitis and pneumonia in ambulatory patients. *Pediatr Inf Dis* 1987; 6: 137-140.

6. Grossman LK, et al: Roentgenographic follow-up of acute pneumonia in children. *Pediatr* 1979; 63: 30-31.

7. Marks MI: Pediatric pneumonia: Viral or bacterial? *J Resp Dis* 1982; 3: 108.

8. McCarthy PL, Frank AL, Ablow RC, et al: Value of the C-reactive protein test in the differentiation of bacterial and viral pneumonias. *Clin Pediatr* 1978; 92: 454-456.

9. McCarthy PL, Spiesel SZ, Stashwick CA, et al: Radiographic findings and etiologic diagnosis in ambulatory childhood pneumonias. *Clin Pediatr* 1981; 20: 686-691.

10. Paisley JW, Lauer BA, Melinkovich P, et al: Rapid diagnosis of chlamydia trachomatis pneumonia in infants by direct immunofluorescence microscopy of nasopharyngeal secretions. *J Pediatr* 1986; 653-654.

11. Paisley JW, Lauer BA, McIntosh K, et al: Pathogens associated with acute lower respiratory tract infections in young children. *Pediatr Inf Dis* 1984; 3: 14-19.

12. Ramsey BWS, Marcuse EK, Fox HM, et al: Use of bacterial antigen detection in the diagnosis of pediatric lower respiratory tract infections. *Pediatr* 1986; 78: 1-9.

13. Tew J, Calenoff L, Berlin BS: Bacterial or nonbacterial pneumonia: Accuracy of radiographic diagnosis. *Radiology* 1977; 124: 607-612.
14. Turner RB, Lande AE, Chase P, et al: Pneumonia in pediatric outpatients: Cause and clinical manifestations. *J Pediatr* 1987; 111: 194-200.
15. Turner RB, Hayden FG, Hendley JO: Etiologic diagnosis of pneumonia in pediatric outpatients by counterimmunoelectrophoresis of urine. *Pediatr* 1983; 71: 780-783.

TRAUMA*

A. Bites - Human

1. Determine circumstances of attack; examine skin carefully.
2. Wash wound immediately; irrigate copiously with sterile saline; debride. Examine for vascular, muscle, tendon, nerve damage.
3. Closed-fist injuries (with wound usually on 1st or 2nd metacarpophalangeal joint) can lead to serious morbidity but may appear benign. Do not suture. Joint infection is one of the main concerns.
4. Use of prophylactic antibiotics in human bites is controversial. Bacteria that cause infections include strep, staph, anaerobes, and rarely aerobic gram-negative organisms. Augmentin (or other penicillinase-resistant antibiotic) will be effective in most of these infections. Continued cleansing must be done at home.
5. Frequent follow-up q 1-3 d to check for infection is advisable.

B. Bites - Animal

1. Determine circumstances of attack, type of animal, whether the animal is domestic or wild, known to victim, current on its rabies shots.

*Contributing author: M. Douglas Baker, M.D., Division of Pediatric Emergency Medicine, Children's Hospital of Philadelphia.

2. Wash the wound (may use Zephiran); irrigate lacerations and deeper wounds with sterile saline; debride thoroughly; examine for vascular, muscle, nerve, tendon damage.

3. Most lacerations can be sutured after cleansing and debridement. Do not suture puncture wounds or small wounds on hand (high risk of infection).

4. Prophylactic antibiotics controversial. Prophylactic Augmentin may be of value in hard-to-irrigate wounds. Bacteria commonly found in infected bites include <u>Pasteurella multocida,</u> strep, and staph. Augmentin will be effective in most cases. Don't forget tetanus prophylaxis.

5. Frequent follow-up q 1-3 d is advisable.

C. Rabies Prophylaxis

1. Rabies is very unusual in domestic cats and dogs.

2. It is also unusual in rodents (rats, squirrels, hamsters, mice) and lagomorphs (rabbits).

3. Most human rabies comes from contact with carnivorous wild animals (skunks, raccoons, foxes) and bats.

4. Unprovoked bites are more likely than provoked to indicate animal is rabid. Bites on a person attempting to feed or handle an apparently healthy animal should generally be regarded as provoked.

5. Outside of caves and laboratories, rabies is transmitted only by introducing the virus into open cuts or wounds in skin, or via mucous membranes.

6. RABIES POSTEXPOSURE GUIDE (Reference - CDC, March, 1980, and Maryland Department of Health and Mental Hygiene, April 1984):
   The following recommendations are only a guide. In applying them, take into account the animal species involved; the circumstances of the bite or other exposure (i.e., scratches, abrasions, open wounds or mucous membranes contaminated with saliva or other potentially infectious material from

a rabid animal); the vaccination status of the animal; and presence of rabies in the region.

	Animal Species	Condition of Animal At Time of Attack	Treatment of Exposed Person*
Domestic	Dog and cat	Healthy and available for 10 days of observation	None, unless animal develops rabies
		Rabid or suspected rabid	RIG and HDCV (see below)
		Unknown (escaped)	Consult public health officials.If treatment is indicated, give RIG and HDCV.
Wild	Skunk, bat, fox coyote, raccoon bobcat, and other carnivores	Regard as rabid unless proved negative by laboratory tests	RIG and HDCV
Other	Livestock, rodents, and lagomorphs (rabbits and hares)	Consider individually. Local and state public health officials should be consulted on questions about the need for rabies prophylaxis. Bites of squirrels, hamsters, guinea pigs, gerbils, chipmunks, rats, mice, other rodents, rabbits, and hares almost never call for antirabies prophylaxis.	

RIG - rabies immune globulin, human
HDCV - human diploid cell vaccine

7. If antirabies treatment is indicated, both RIG and HDCV should be given as soon as possible, regardless of the interval from exposure.
8. Dose of RIG: 20 IU/kg
   a. If possible, infiltrate half the dose around the wound and give the rest IM.
   b. RIG provides passive immunity while body mounts active immune response.
   c. If RIG was not given when vaccination was begun, it can be given up to the 8th day after the first dose of vaccine was given. Thereafter RIG is unnecessary, since presumably an active antibody response to the vaccine has occurred.
9. Dose of HDCV: Five 1 cc doses, IM
   a. HDCV induces an active immune response that requires about 7-10 days to develop, but persists for as long as 1 yr.

   b. Give first dose as soon as possible after exposure, additional doses 3, 7, 14, and 28 days after the first dose.
   c. A serum specimen for rabies antibody testing is no longer necessary unless the patient is suspected of being immunocompromised, i.e., receiving steroids or immunosuppressive therapy that is essential for the treatment of another condition.

10. Side effects
    a. HDCV - Side effects less frequent than with the duck embryo vaccine used formerly. Local reactions: pain, erythema, swelling or itching in 25% of recipients. Systemic: headache, nausea, abdominal pain, muscle aches and dizziness in 20%. No serious anaphylactic, systemic, or neuroparalytic reactions have been reported. Once rabies prophylaxis is started, don't interrupt or discontinue it because of local or mild systemic reactions. Usually these reactions can be managed with acetaminophen.
    b. RIG - Much better than old equine antirabies serum. Fever or localized pain most common side effects.

11. If patient bitten by dog, give parents instruction on wound care. Ask parents to report bite to police. The dog must be watched for 10 days by owners or dog pound for signs of rabies.

12. Give tetanus prophylaxis if indicated.

D. Burns

1. Children with first degree burns (erythema only) may be treated with analgesics, cool compresses, suntan creams, and, if itching is a problem, oral antihistamines.

2. Children with second degree burns (painful, blisters, ± areas of blanching within the burn area) may need to be hospitalized if the total body surface burned is (a) >5% in infants, (b) >10% in chil-

dren, (c) >15% in adolescents/adults, and (d) burns involving the face, perineum, hands, and feet.

   a. The initial management of second degree burns includes cleansing the area with saline, trimming broken blisters or ragged skin edges (leaving intact blisters alone), applying 1% silver sulfadiazine (Silvadene) or Xeroform to a more superficial burn, securing burn with clean gauze (and a stockette if necessary for the particular body part).

   b. The patient should be seen daily until healing is well under way. Further debridement, if necessary, can be done at these visits.

   c. Burn cleansing and dressing may be done at home, but the Silvadene must be completely removed before each cleansing and redressing.

   d. At the first signs of burn infection (redness of edges, purulence), systemic antibiotics should be instituted.

   e. Pain relief should be provided by analgesics (acetaminophen, codeine); Parenteral narcotics may be more useful than oral agents in hospitalized patients.

   f. Once the burn has healed (7-14 d), an emollient should be applied to protect the new, fragile epidermis; protection against strong sunlight should also be instituted.

3. For the management of children with extensive second degree or third degree burns, see *Harriet Lane Handbook* pp. 225-8.

E. Dental Trauma

1. There are various types of dental trauma:

   a. Concussion: injury to periodontal ligaments without displacement or mobility of the tooth; there is percussion sensitivity.

   b. Subluxation: tooth is mobile horizontally and is tender to percussion.

    c. Displacement: tooth is intruded into socket, extruded lingually, or avulsed.

    d. Fracture: in enamel fracture, only an edge is missing; in crown fractures, there are cracks in the enamel but there is no tooth discoloration; in dentin fractures, there is a yellow discoloration (if the pulp is exposed, a pinkish color is obvious).

    e. Mandibular fracture: unilateral-mandible deviates toward affected side; bilateral-mouth is gaping and malocclusion is present.

    f. Maxillary fracture: involvement of bony processes into which teeth are imbedded; teeth may be displaced and mobile.

2. Examine the face and lips for obvious traumatic lesions and asymmetries.

    a. The mandible and maxilla should be palpated for tenderness.

    b. The patient should open and close his mouth so that asymmetrical and unstable areas may be appreciated.

    c. The mouth should be examined for bleeding, swelling, or broken teeth.

    d. With the patient biting down, ask if his bite feels normal.

    e. Check each tooth individually for pain and mobility.

3. Concussions, crown and enamel fractures require elective dental referral.

    a. Other conditions listed above in #1 (b, c, d) require immediate dental referral.

    b. Fractures of the upper or lower jaw require an oral surgeon.

    d. An avulsed permanent tooth may be reimplanted within an hour of the injury; do not reimplant primary teeth.

F. **Frostbite**

1. In frostbite, freezing of tissues occurs.

a. The toes, fingers, ears, and nose are commonly involved.

b. Initially, the frostbitten tissue is white, firm and numb; with progression, cyanosis, mottling, and vesicles appear.

c. On rewarming, superficially frostbitten areas become red, swollen, and painful; no cyanosis is present and sensation is normal.

d. On rewarming, deeply frostbitten areas may be cyanotic, lack sensation, and be excrutiatingly painful.

2. Treatment is by rapidly warming affected areas in tepid water (105°-110° F) for 20-40 minutes.

a. Do not rub (increases tissue injury).

b. If vesicles or bullae are present, do not rupture but, instead, cover them with gauze.

c. Plastic surgery consultation and hospitalization are necessary whenever there is deep frostbite.

G. Insect Reactions

1. The reaction to insect bites or stings may be local (redness, pain, swelling at the site) and/or systemic (urticaria, hypotension, wheezing, laryngeal edema, shock); these reactions generally occur within 2 hours of the sting.

a. Delayed reactions can occur up to a week following the sting and include fever, arthralgias, urticaria and rarely, neuritis or vasculitis.

b. Always try to identify the stinging insect by history and to determine if there have been previous systemic (or local) reactions to stings or if there is a history of allergy.

2. Treatment for local reactions include stinger removal, cleansing and applying ice to the area, and Benadryl (5 mg/kg/d ÷ qid).

a. If the wound is >24 hours old and seems infected (tumor, rubor, dolor, calor), dicloxacillin (40-50 mg/kg/d ÷ qid) should be given.

b. For mild systemic reactions (e.g., generalized

urticaria) occurring immediately, Benadryl (5 mg/kg/d ÷ qid) or Atarax (2 mg/kg/d ÷ qid) may be given.

c. For anaphylactic reactions, epinephrine (0.01 cc/kg of 1: 1000 concentration) is given SQ and locally; a tourniquet should be placed above the site. The patient may require IV fluids, aminophylline (6 mg/kg bolus), hydrocortisone (10 mg/kg), and intubation.

H. Ticks and Spiders

1. The tick attaches itself to the skin; its saliva can induce tissue destruction. It should be promptly removed by applying steady, slow traction with forceps (or at home, tweezers). Don't squeeze the tick or crush it. If the tick's mouth parts remain after removal, an ulcer or granuloma may develop; intralesional steroids or excision treats the lesion.

2. Ticks spread Rocky Mountain Spotted Fever (relapsing fever, headache) and Lyme disease (erythema chronicum migrans, polyarthritis, neurologic disease, carditis).
   Treatment of RMSF is tetracycline 25-40 mg/kg q 6 h (max = 2g/day) or IV chloramphenicol 50-100 mg/kg/d (max. 4g/d). Try to keep near 50 to decrease likelihood of chloramphenicol toxicity. Treatment of Lyme disease is Penicillin G 250,000 units qid x 7-10 d (alternative is tetracycline).

3. Spiders - Black widow spiders produce a neurotoxin that causes severe muscular cramps and pain and a rigid abdomen within a half-hour after the bite.
   a. Muscle spasms may be relieved by diazepam 5-10 mg and intravenous calcium gluconate.
   b. The neurotoxin may also cause an ascending motor paralysis; fever, vomiting, convulsions and shock may occur.
   c. A specific antivenom (Lyovac) is useful for high-risk patients who test negative for allergy to horse serum.

      d. Narcotics may be necessary for pain relief.

4. The bites of brown recluse spiders induce, in mild cases, redness and swelling at the site; in moderate to severe cases, there is local tissue and vessel damage and necrosis and systemic reactions such as a generalized rash, urticaria, arthralgias, fever, nausea, vomiting, and occasionally, hemolysis or DIC.

5. The bites of other spiders cause pain, swelling, pruritis at the site.

6. Tetanus prophylaxis is advisable after any spider bite.

7. Treatment for local reactions consists of Benadryl or Atarax.

8. Systemic steroids are indicated for patients with systemic symptoms or with bites in cosmetic or functional areas. In these patients, monitoring for the onset of hemolysis or DIC is mandatory.

    Plastic surgery is usually necessary for a good cosmetic result in the bite area.

I. Lacerations

1. Determine how the injury happened, how long ago, and where (outdoors, home, etc.); the patient's last tetanus shot; other medical problems and medications.

2. Calm the patient and family. Parents may help to comfort the child by staying nearby.

3. Test function of muscle, tendon, nerve, and vascular status before anesthesia. Thoroughly examine wound. If it appears complicated or deep, call surgeon.

4. Sterile technique is mandatory. Wash hands; apply sterile gloves.

5. Place drainage pad under wound.

6. Swab surrounding skin with Betadine.

7. Administer local anesthesia.

    a. Use 1% xylocaine with 25 gauge needle.

    b. May use 1% xylocaine with epinephrine on face or scalp to decrease bleeding, but never on fingers or toes.

    c. Always aspirate before injection to avoid IV injection.

    d. A new local anesthestic method, TAC (tetracaine, adrenaline, and cocaine) applied via saturated gauze, is showing great promise.

8. After lesion is anesthetized, irrigate <u>copiously</u> with saline and drain adequately.

9. Explore wound for deep injury. Remove foreign bodies and dirt. Scrub when necessary.

10. Obtain x-ray of wound if <u>any</u> suspicion of residual metal pieces or glass. Metal and glass will show on x-ray. Wood and plastic will not.

11. Suture: NOTE: Needle size - as # increases, radius increases.
                    Suture size - as # of 0's increase, caliber decreases.

    a. 5-0 or 6-0 nylon on hands and face; 4-0 elsewhere, except 3-0 nylon for scalp and knee lacerations on older children.

    b. 4-0, 3-0, or 2-0 absorbable (Vicryl) sutures for subcutaneous sutures.

    c. Avoid dead space (i.e., close it).

12. Apply dressing:

    a. Dress in position for function.

    b. Apply antibiotic ointment.

    c. Cover with 4 x 4s or similar material, 2-3 inches beyond wound edge. For burns and abrasions, use a non-adhesive dressing such as Xeroform.

    d. Apply "Kling" if needed. Also, may use fluffed cotton.

    e. Benzoin tincture for tape adhesion.

    f. Ace bandage occasionally neeeded for immobilization or hemostasis.

13. Immobilization is sometimes required if laceration is in mobile area. Continue splint 1-2 wk after sutures out.

14. Advise elevation x 24 h for lacerations involving hands and feet to avoid edema.
15. How long to keep sutures in:
    a. Face: 4-5 d; then may steristrip.
    b. Non-mobile area; 5-7 d; then may steristrip.
    c. Distal site or mobile area; 7-14 d; then may steristrip.
16. Give tetanus prophylaxis, if needed.
17. Antibiotic not generally used unless laceration is very dirty (e.g., human bite).
18. When/When <u>not</u> to suture:
    a. Ideally, wounds should be sutured within 8 hours.
    b. Puncture wounds are usually closed by the time the child presents for medical attention. If so, clean thoroughly with Betadine; do not reopen. If the wound is slightly open, clean with Saline and irrigate copiously. <u>Never</u> suture a puncture wound (increased risk of infection).
    c. Up to 24 hours, you can approximate wound with steristrips or loose sutures, but <u>only after</u> laceration is thoroughly cleansed and irrigated.

REFERENCES

Bites - Human
1. Baker MD: Human bites in children. *AJDC* 1987; 141: 1285-90.
2. Brook I: Microbiology of human and animal bite wounds. *Pediatr Infect Dis* 1987; 6: 29-32.
3. Schweich P, Fleisher G: Human bites in children. *Pediatr Emerg Care* 1985; 1: 51-3.

Bites - Animal
1. Boenning D, et al: Dog bites in children. *Am J Emerg Med* 1983; 1: 17-21.
2. Brook I: Microbiology of human and animal bite wounds in children. *Pediatr Infec Dis* 1987; 6: 29-32.
3. Feder H, et al: Review of 59 patients hospitalized with animal bites. *Pediatr Infect Dis* 1987; 6: 24-28.
4. Marcy SM: Infections due to dog and cat bites. *Pediatr Infect Dis* 1982; 1: 351-6.
5. Trott A: Care of mammalian bites. *Pediatr Infect Dis* 1987; 6: 8-10.

Rabies Prophylaxis
1. Rabies Prevention. *Morbidity and Mortality Weekly Report* 1980; 29: 265-80.
2. Kaplan MM, Koprowski H: Rabies. *Scientific American* 1980 242: 120-131, 1980.
3. Mann J: Systemic decision-making in rabies prophylaxis. *Pediatr Infect Dis* 1983; 2: 162-7.
4. Maryland Department of Health and Mental Hygiene - Preventive Medicine Administration: Rabies Prevention in Maryland, April 1984, p. 1-12.

Burns
1. Coren C: Burn injuries in children. *Pediatr Ann* 1987; 16: 328-39.
2. Fitzpatrick K, et al: Outpatient management of minor burns. *Physic Asst* 1985; 16-28.
3. Gellis S, Kagan B: Current Pediatric Therapy - 12. Philadelphia: WB Saunders Co., 1986; pp. 685-7.
4. Guzzetta P, Randolph J: Burns in children.1982. *Pediatr in Rev* 1983; 4: 271-9.

5. Robinson M, Seward P: Thermal injury in children. *Pediatr Emerg Care* 1987; 3: 266-70.

6. Herndon Dm, Thompson PB, Desai MH, et al: Treatment of burns in children. *Pediatr Clin N Am* 1985; 32: 1311-1332.

Dental Trauma

1. Berkowitz R, et al: Dental trauma in children and adolescents. *Clin Pediatr* 1980; 19: 166-71.

2. Committee on Early Childhood, Adoption, and Dependent Care: Oral and dental aspects of child abuse and neglect. *Pediatr* 1986; 78: 537-9.

3. McTigue D: Management of orofacial trauma in children. *Pediatr Ann* 1985; 14: 125-9.

Frostbite

1. Paton B: A quick, effective response to hypothermia and frostbite. *Contemp Pediatr* 1986; 3: 37-52.

Insect reactions

1. Goldberg G: Stings and bites - emergencies and annoyances. *Contemp Pediatr* 1985; 2: 32-46.

2. Maguire J, Geha R: Bee, wasp, and hornet stings. *Pediatr in Rev* 1986; 8: 5-11.

Ticks & Spiders

1. Goldberg G: Stings and bites - emergencies and annoyances. *Contemp Pediatri* 1985; 2: 32-46.

Lacerations

1. Bonadio W, Wagner V: Efficacy of TAC topical anesthetic for Repair of pediatric lacerations. *AJDC* 1988; 142: 203-5.

19

SEXUALLY TRANSMITTED DISEASES

A. General

Clinical presentation may include urethritis, vulvovaginitis, cervicitis, dysuria in women, inguinal lymphadenopathy, pelvic inflammatory disease (PID), epididymitis, proctitis, pharyngitis, arthritis, conjunctivitis, and ulcerations on penis, vulva, or vagina.

At least 20 different causative microorganisms are now recognized (bacteria, viruses, fungi, protozoans, arthropods). Some of these are:

B. Gonorrhea

1. May be seen at any age. If prepubertal, suspect sexual abuse.
2. May be asymptomatic (>50% females; 25% males).
3. Culture cervix, urethra, pharynx, rectum, and inflamed joint if index of suspicion is high.
4. Diagnosis
   a. Gram stain showing >8 gram-negative intracellular diplococci (more reliable on urethral swab of male; less reliable on endocervical swab of female). Confirm with culture.
   b. Send specimen to lab for culture immediately.

5. Screen for syphilis on all patients suspected of having GC (VDRL, STS). Consider other sexually transmitted infections (HSV, Chlamydia, Trichomonas, etc.).

6. Treatment (current recommendations reflect the increase in penicillinase-producing strains)
   a. Asymptomatic and uncomplicated Gonorrhea infections (vaginitis, cervicitis, urethritis, proctitis, pharyngitis)
      1) Ceftriaxone 125-250 mg IM once
         alternative
      2) 1 gm probenecid po, with 3.5 ampicillin po or 3.0 gm amoxicillin po. (This regimen should not be used if pharyngeal or anorectal GC is suspected or for penicillinase-producing N. gonorrhoeae).
      3) Spectinomycin 2 gm IM is an alternative for rectal, urethral, or cervical GC.
      4) None of these regimens treats Chlamydia. Always treat for Chlamydia when treating for GC. (See page 286.)
      5) Prepubertal children (>45 kg)
         a) Ceftriaxone 125 mg IM once.
         b) Probenecid 25 mg/kg (maximum 1.0 g) po followed by 100,000 units/kg procaine penicillin IM or amoxicillin 50 mg/kg po once.
         c) Spectinomycin 40 mg/kg IM once.
            NOTE: Follow-up culture is mandatory. Obtain it about 1 week after treatment is completed. Don't forget to treat contacts.
   b. Disseminated Gonococcal Infections (DGI)-symptoms include dermatitis and arthritis.
      1) Ceftriaxone 1g IV qd x 7 d.
      2) IV Penicillin G 10 million units/d for minimum of 3 days, followed by po ampicillin 500 mg qid x 4d.
      3) Doxycycline 100 mg po bid x 7d.

C. PID (salpingitis)

1. Fever in only 33% of patients. Patients may have lower abdominal pain, vaginal discharge, irregular bleeding, cervical motion/adnexal tenderness. Risk of subsequent sterility exists. Remove IUD if present.

2. Etiology: Often polymicrobial. Most frequent pathogens are <u>N. gonorrhoeae</u>, and anaerobic bacteria (most commonly <u>Peptostreptococcus, Peptococcus, Bacteroides</u> species). Other organisms include <u>Mycoplasma hominis, Ureaplasma urealyticum,</u> and <u>Chlamydia trachomatis.</u>

3. Hospitalize if:
   a. Uncertain diagnosis.
   b. Surgical emergencies such as ectopic pregnancy and appendicitis are to be R/O'd.
   c. High suspicion of pelvic abscess.
   d. Severe illness (T>101; wbc >20,000).
   e. Patient is pregnant.
   f. Patient cannot follow outpatient regimen, cannot tolerate po medications or cannot come back for F/U in 48-72 h.
   g. Patient has not responded to outpatient Rx.

4. Treatment
   a. Outpatient:
      1) Cefoxitin 2 g IM once and probenicid 1g po once.
      2) Ceftriaxone 250 mg IM once.
      3) <u>Both</u> 1) and 2) should be followed by Doxycycline 100 mg po bid x 10d.
   b. If hospitalized (GYN may be consulted):
      1) Cefoxitin 2 g IV qid plus Doxycycline 100 mg IV bid until improvement, followed by Doxycycline 100 mg po bid to complete 10d course.
      2) Alternative is clindamycin 600 mg IV qid plus gentamycin 2 mg/kg IV once followed by Gentamycin 1.5 mg/kg IV tid until improvement followed by clindamycin 450 mg po qid to complete 10-14 d course.

       c. Miscellaneous
         1) Treat contacts.
         2) Get follow-up culture.

D. Fitzhugh-Curtis Syndrome: extension of infection from salpingitis to capsule and outer surface of liver. Consider if patient presents with RUQ pain, palpable liver, abnormal LFTs or adnexal/cervical motion tenderness. Treatment is as under 4b.

E. Chlamydial Infections

1. May be found in mixed infections.
2. May present with urethritis, cervicitis, dysuria in females, salpingitis, inguinal lymphadenopathy, Fitzhugh-Curtis syndrome, epididymitis, proctitis; may be asymptomatic.
3. Diagnosis: Culture in specific media; microtrak (direct fluorescent staining); ELISA; endocervical Gram stain >10 wbcs per oil immersion field; in males >10 wbcs per hpf in 1st 15cc of void.
4. Treatment
   a. Doxycycline 100 mg po bid x 7d (not in pregnancy).
   b. Erythromycin 500 mg qid x 7 d.
   c. Sulfisoxazole 500 mg qid x 10 d.
5. Be sure to contact and treat sexual partners.

F. Syphilis

1. Forms
   a. Congenital form: mucocutaneous lesions, "snuffles" rash, bone changes (painful, pseudoparalysis, dactylitis), hepatosplenomegaly, lymphadenopathy, fever, anemia, FTT. Infants may not always manifest symptoms.
     1) Infected infants may be sero-negative if maternal infection was late in gestation.
     2) Infants should be treated at birth if maternal treatment was inadequate, unknown, or with drugs other than penicillin, or if adequate F/U cannot be assured.

   3) Always examine CSF before treatment.
  b. Acquired syphilis: primary stage: chancre detectable in adolescents and adults, less common in children. Secondary stage: rash, condylomata lata.
2. Evaluation
  a. Serology for VDRL or FT-ABS.
  b. CSF - protein, cells, VDRL or FT-ABS, do dark-field exam for spirochetes.
  c. Scrape any mucosal, cutaneous lesion and do dark-field exam.
  d. X-rays as indicated for congenital form.
3. Treatment
  a. Congenital syphilis without CNS involvement: Benzathine Pen G 50,000 units/kg IM single dose. With CNS involvement: Procaine Pen G 50,000 units/kg/d IM or IV x 10-14d. If CSF is initially positive, reexamine CSF q 6 months until normal. Repeat if CSF serology test remains positive for 6 mo after first therapy, if blood serology remains positive 1 yr after Rx, or if 4-fold rise in VDRL.
  b. Acquired syphilis
    1) For primary, secondary, or early latent syphilis (<1 yr duration) Benzathine Pencillin G 2.4 million units IM in a single dose.
       Alternate therapy if penicillin absolutely cannot be used: Erythromycin or tetracycline (> 8 yr old) both 500 mg qid po x 15 d.
       Need follow-up serology: Successful if negative serology in primary syphilis by 12 mo; in secondary syphilis by 24 mo; in latent syphilis by 48 mo.
    2) For syphilis >1 yr duration: Benzathine Pen G 2.4 million units IM every 7d x 3 wk. (Total 7.2 million units); alternatively, tetracycline or erythromycin, 500 mg qid x 30 days. Repeat if there is not a 4-fold decrease in titer by 1 yr after Rx or if clinical s/sx persist.

by 1 yr after Rx or if clinical s/sx persist.
REMEMBER: Contact, evaluate, and treat all sexual partners.

3) For neurosyphilis: Penicillin G 2.4 million units IV q 4 h x 10d or Penicillin G 2.4 million units IM qd plus probenecid 500 mg qid x 10 d, either regimen followed by Penicillin G benzathine 2.4 million units IM weekly x 3 weeks.

4) F/U and Retreatment
   a) All patients with early syphilis and congenital syphilis should have repeat VDRLs at 3, 6, and 12 months after treatment.
   b) The VDRL will be non-reactive or reactive with a low titer within a year following successful therapy.
   c) The possibility of reinfection should be considered when a patient with early syphilis needs to be retreated. Retreatment should be considered when:
      (1) Clinical signs of syphilis persist or recur.
      (2) There is a 4-fold increase in VDRL titre.
      (3) A high titre VDRL fails to show a 4-fold decrease in one year. Retreat according to schedules recommended for syphilis of more than one year's duration.

G. Herpes Simplex Virus

1. Patient may be asymptomatic or have painful ulcerations on genitalia; ulcers between vaginal folds and posterior cervix can be easily missed.
   a. Cytology (e.g., Pap smear or Tsanck stain) will reveal multinucleated giant cells in ~75% of culture positive specimens.
   b. Viral medium is needed for culture.
2. Treatment: acyclovir ointment 5% (Zovirax) indicated in management of <u>initial</u> (not recurrent) herpes genitalis. Apply sufficient quantity to cover all lesions q 3 h, 6 times per d x 7 d. A finger cot or

glove should be used when applying ointment to prevent autoinoculation of other body sites or transmission to other people. Acyclovir will decrease viral shedding and duration of pain.

H. Hepatitis B

1. Clinically: jaundice, anorexia, vomiting, liver enlargement/tenderness, etc.
2. Chemistries: ↑ LFTs and ↑ bilirubin; +serology for hepatitis B. If severe liver disease, PT/PTT may be prolonged.
3. Abnormal U/A (↑ bilirubin); abnormal stool (acholic)
4. Preventive measures: see page 143.

I. Condylomata Acuminata

1. This type of wart is caused by the human papilloma virus; the incubation period is weeks. Certain types are associated with genital neoplasia.
2. The wart has a cauliflower (white or strawberry pink-red) appearance and can be located on the genitalia, around the anus, or in and around the mouth. At the time of detection, the lesions may range in size from several mm to several cm due to confluence of multiple lesions.
3. Physical exam and laboratory tests are necessary to R/O other veneral diseases.
4. Treatment is by careful application of 3% tincture of podophyllin to external lesions on a weekly basis.
   a. Podophyllin should not be used for internal lesions.
   b. The medication should be left on for 2-4 h and then washed off with warm soap and water.
   c. Surrounding skin areas should be protected with petroleum jelly during podophyllin application.
5. Recalcitrant warts and those in the urethra, vagina, or rectum may require cryotherapy with liquid N_2 or laser surgery.

J. Human Immunodeficiency Virus (HIV)

1. Suspect this agent if a patient presents with fever, weight loss, respiratory symptoms, and lymphadenopathy. Seek a history of anal intercourse, IV drug use, blood transfusions, or sexual contact with an HIV positive person. Infants and toddlers can present with failure to thrive; seek a history of maternal HIV infection.

2. Initial testing for HIV is done via an ELISA test. If the test is negative, no further tests are necessary. If the ELISA result is questionable or positive, the Western Blot test is then run.

3. Repeat testing after several months may be necessary.

4. Vaccine and AZT trials are underway. Currently, there is no cure for HIV infection.

REFERENCES

General

1. Bell T: Major sexually transmitted diseases of children and adolescents. *Pediatr Infec Dis* 1983; 2:153-61.
2. Farmer M, et al: Laboratory evaluation of sexually transmitted diseases. *Pediatr Ann* 1986; 15:715-24.
3. Frau L, Alexander ER: Public health implications of sexually transmitted disease in pediatric practice. *Pediatr Infect Dis* 1985; 4:453-67.
4. Martien K, Emans SJ: Treatment of common genital infections in adolescents. *J Adol Hth Care* 1987; 8:129-36.
5. Sexually Transmitted Diseases - Treatment Guidelines 1982. *MMWR Supplement.* 8/20/82; Vol 31, #25.
6. Treatment of Sexually Transmitted Diseases. *The Medical Letter* 2/28/86; Vol 28, #708.

Gonorrhea

1. Whittington W, et al: Incorrect identification of N. Gonorrhea from infants & children. *Pediatr Infect Dis* 1988; 7:3-10.

Chlamydial Infections

1. Bell T, et al: Delayed appearance of Chlamydia trachomatis infections acquired at birth. *Pediatr Infect Dis* 1987; 6:928-31.
2. Hammerschlag M: Infections due to Chlamydia trachomatis. *Pediatr Ann* 1984; 13:673-82.
3. McMillan J: Chlaymdia - unsuspected, undiagnosed, untreated. *Contemp Pediatr* 1985; 2:14-28.
4. Rettig P: Chlamydial infections in pediatrics - Diagnostic and therapeutic considerations. *Pediatr Infect Dis* 1986; 5:158-62.
5. Rettig P: Infections due to Chlamydia trachomatis from infancy to adolescence. *Pediatr Infect Dis* 1986; 5:449-57.

Syphilis

1. Ginsburg C: Acquired syphilis in prepubertal children. *Pediatr Infect Dis* 1983; 2:232-4.
2. Pickering L: Diagnosis and therapy of patients with congenital & primary syphilis. *Pediatr Infect Dis* 1985; 4:602-5.
3. Srinivasan G, et al: Congenital syphilis - a diagnostic and therapeutic dilemma. *Pediatr Infect Dis* 1983; 2:436-41.

Herpes Simplex Virus
1. Bryson Y: The use of acyclovir in children. *Pediatr Infect Dis* 1984; 3:345-8.
2. Bryson Y, et al: Treatment of first episodes of genital herpes simplex virus infection with oral acyclovir. *NEJM* 1983; 308:916-21.
3. Corey L: The diagnosis and treatment of genital herpes. *JAMA* 1982; 248:1041-9.
4. Douglas J, et al: A double-blind study of oral acyclovir for suppression of recurrences of genital herpes simplex virus infection. *NEJM* 1984; 310:1551-56.
5. Solomon A, et al: The Tzanck smear in the diagnosis of cutaneous herpes simplex. *JAMA* 1984; 251:633-5.
6. Straus S, et al: Suppression of frequently recurring genital herpes. *NEJM* 1984; 310:1545-50.
7. Whitley R, Alford C: Herpes virus Infections in childhood - diagnostic dilemmas and therapy. *Pediatr Infect Dis* 1982; 1:81-4.

Hepatitis B
1. Committee on Infectious Diseases: Prevention of hepatitis B virus infections. *Pediatr* 1985; 75:362-4.
2. Forster J: Best Prevention measures for hepatitis B. *Contemp Pediatr* 1984; 1:37-45.
3. Inactivated hepatitis B virus vaccine. *MMWR* 6/25/82, Vol 31, #24.
4. Pickering L: Management of the infant of a mother with viral hepatitis. *Pediatr in Rev* 1988; 9:315-20.

Human Immunodeficiency Virus
1. Ammann A, Shannon K: Recognition of acquired immune deficiency syndrome (AIDS) in children. *Pediatr in Rev* 1985; 7:101-8.
2. Barrett D: The clinician's guide to pediatric AIDS. *Contemp Pediatr* 1988; 5:24-47.
3. CDC: Recommendations for prevention of HIV transmission in health-care settings. *MMWR Supplement* 8/21/87; Vol 36, #2S.

4. Ochs H: Intravenous immunoglobulin in the treatment and prevention of acute infections in pediatric acquired immunodeficiency syndrome patients. *Pediatr Infect Dis* 1987; 6:509-11.
5. Oleske J, et al: Treatment of HIV infected infants and children. *Pediatr Ann* 1988; 17:332-7.
6. Rogers M: Pediatric HIV infection. *Pediatr Ann* 1988; 17:324-31.
7. Scott G: Clinical manifestations of HIV infection in children. *Pediatr Ann* 1988; 17:365-9.

20

MISCELLANEOUS

A. Chest Pain

1. Chest pain is a relatively infrequent presenting complaint in young children but becomes more frequent as children age. It can be functional, herald serious disease, or have a significance somewhere in between.
2. Important historical information includes
   a. The pain's onset, duration, recurrence, location, radiation, quality (sharp vs dull),
   b. Relationship of pain to rest, exercise, and eating,
   c. Precipitating factors,
   d. Actions or medications that make the pain improve,
   e. Previous history of similar pain or being awakened from sleep by pain,
   f. Other concomitant symptoms (diaphoresis, nausea, vomiting, dyspnea, coughing, wheezing, vertigo, syncope, palpitations, skin color changes),
   g. Presence of fever, respiratory symptoms, and myalgias (especially if pain is acute),
   h. Symptoms of indigestion,
   i. The possibility of foreign body aspiration,
   j. A history of trauma,

      k. A past history of a heart murmur, cardiac disease or surgery, sickle cell disease, chronic respiratory disease,

      l. Psychosomatic symptoms (is child under stress),

      m. Medication or illicit drug use,

      n. Family history of angina, cardiac disease, death (especially if recent) from cardiac causes.

3. The physical exam should be complete with special emphasis on

    a. Vital signs,

    b. General appearance (frightened, in pain, indifferent, etc.),

    c. Skin (cyanosis, pallor),

    d. Respiratory exam (rate, depth, symmetry of respirations, splinting, rales, wheezes, areas of decreased breath sounds),

    e. Cardiac exam (PMI, rate, regularity of rhythm, murmurs, rubs, gallops, assessment of pulse equality and strength, palpation of chest and neck for thrills, auscultation of neck for bruits); remember to auscultate in both supine and sitting positions.

    f. The chest wall (areas of tenderness, asymmetry, inflammation, whether direct palpation reproduces pain, palpation of ribs, intercostal spaces, upper abdomen, and vertebral bodies to determine direct or referred areas of tenderness).

4. Causes of chest pain

    a. Cardiac (suggested by pain associated with exercise, palpitations, color changes, syncope, vertigo).

      1) Ischemia (squeezing pain, tachypnea, tachycardia, gallop, rales, wheezes, CHF, shock).

      2) Left Ventricular Outflow Obstruction (especially precipitated by exercise when cardiac oxygen demand is not met by its supply): aortic valve or subvalvular stenosis (harsh systolic murmurs varying little with ma-

neuvers altering ventricular filling), idiopathic hypertrophic subaortic stenosis (murmur softens during valsalva; pansystolic murmur with S_4; ECG <u>may</u> show septal Q wave).

3) Coronary artery disease (compression, fistula, secondary to collagen-vascular disease or mucocutaneous lymph node syndrome): systolic/continuous murmur, gallop; ECG may show infarction or ST-T wave changes.

4) Mitral valve prolapse (usually asymptomatic): mid-systolic click and/or late systolic murmur (altered by position); ECG may show T wave changes, U wave, tachycardia.

5) Dissecting aortic aneurysm (acute, sharp, "tearing" pain - emergency).

6) Arrhythmias (may have palpitations, chest pain, dizziness): may be tachycardia, bradycardia, or varying rhythms.

7) Pericardial infection, inflammation, or infiltration by tumor (sharp pain exacerbated by inspiration, cough, movement): friction rub heard on auscultation; ECG may show ST elevation and low QRS voltage.

b. Pulmonary

1) Pneumonia (rales, decreased breath sounds, tachypnea, cough, respiratory distress).

2) Asthma.

3) Pleurisy (sharp pain aggravated by cough/inspiration).

4) Pneumothorax (sharp pain peripherally, dyspnea, areas of decreased breath sounds).

5) Pulmonary infarction (intense pain, respiratory distress, may be cyanosis and shock).

c. Gastrointestinal

1) Esophageal reflux (substernal pain, which is worse after eating or when supine); aerophagia; belching.

2) Esophagitis (similar pain as in reflux but may be more intense).

3) Hiatal hernia.
4) Mallory-Weiss syndrome (acute onset).
5) Gastric spasm, inflammation, ulcer (lower chest, epigastric pain elicited by direct palpation).
6) Duodenal ulcer.
7) Biliary/pancreatic disease.

d. Mediastinal diseases (pneumomediastinum, tumors, mediastinitis.)

e. Chest Wall Disorders
   1) Costochondritis (tender costochondral junctions).
   2) Trauma (may reproduce pain with palpation over affected area).
   3) Breast development.

f. Emotional (pain vague, fleeting, localized over heart or left arm, not precipitated by exercise, may be at rest, other psychosomatic symptoms may be present).

g. Precordial Catch Syndrome (sharp pain below left sternal border or left breast without radiation; it is relieved by change of position, chest massage, or deep inspiration).

h. Miscellaneous (chest wall zoster, malignancies, hemoglobinopathies, collagen vascular diseases, spinal root irritations).

5. Laboratory tests should be dictated by the history and physical findings.
   a. If a cardiac cause for pain is suspected (pain with exercise, palpitations, color changes, syncope, etc.), an ECG, echocardiogram, and/or prompt referral to a cardiologist are in order.
   b. If a pulmonary cause is likely, a chest film may be useful.

6. Treatment is directed to the underlying cause of the chest pain.

B. Failure to Thrive (FTT)

1. FTT is defined as weight <3%ile <u>or</u> <80% of ideal weight <u>or</u> decreasing by at least 2 percentile lines on a growth chart. The height and head circumference usually are not as affected as the weight.
   a. There is an equal race and sex incidence.
   b. Most patients are younger than 24-36 mo of age.
   c. FTT may be the reason for presentation or may be an "incidental" finding when the child presents for an acute illness.

2. Important historical information includes
   a. Prenatal, birth, neonatal histories (especially maternal exposure to drugs, cigarettes, infectious agents),
   b. Sleep, bowel and bladder habits,
   c. Developmental history (age-appropriate; is delay present? is it global or local?),
   d. Feeding history ("average" day diet recall, type of formula used and how it is prepared; amount of formula/milk ingested/day, amount and types of other fluids ingested/day; amount and types of solids ingested/day),
   e. Presence of "meal battles," presence of feeding difficulties-tongue thrusting, choking, diaphoresis, color changes, regurgitation,
   f. How child is fed (can child feed self, drink from a cup),
   g. Presence of infectious disease symptoms (which ones), chronic medical conditions, chronic medication use,
   h. Past history,
   i. Review of systems,
   j. Family history (especially heights/weights of parents, siblings, grandparents),
   k. Social history (child's affect, and behavior; was this child planned?; parental history of abuse or FTT; family's financial and living conditions; parent's social supports; parent's bond with child; other caretakers of child).

3. A complete, meticulous physical examination is <u>mandatory</u>!
   a. Particular attention should be paid to growth parameters; Wt, Ht, HC should be measured and plotted against the child's age.
      1) Wt, Ht, HC all <3%ile - usually in utero insult; however, may be severe, prolonged caloric deprivation.
      2) Wt and Ht <3%ile, HC ok - endocrinopathies, structural dystrophies, constitutional short stature.
      3) Wt <3% ile, Ht and HC ok - caloric deprivation (poor intake vs. poor utilization), nonorganic FTT.
   b. Child's appearance (clean vs. dirty, small vs. scrawny, fearful vs. too trusting, clinging, avoiding mother, avoiding eye-contact).
   c. Skin (dirty, rashes, chronic conditions such as eczema, signs of abuse).
   d. Muscle mass (decreased, with little fat).
   e. Head (asymmetries, overriding/separated sutures, size, shape, texture of fontanelle, flattened or balding occiput, signs of trauma); transilluminate infant's head.
   f. Mouth (tongue thrust, enlarged tongue); teeth (number, condition).
   g. Cardiopulmonary (any abnormality).
   h. Abdomen (organomegaly, protuberance, etc.).
   i. Extremities (length relative to trunk length).
   j. Neurologic/developmental assessment.
4. Causes of FTT
   a. Organic (30-40% of cases)
      1) GI (40% of all organic FTTs): most commonly clefts, chalasia, gastroesophageal reflux, celiac disease, Crohn's, Hirschsprung's, cystic fibrosis, liver disease
      2) Renal: remember renal tubular acidosis in addition to more obvious diseases.
      3) CNS (20% of all organic FTTs).

       4) Endocrine: diabetes mellitus, diabetes insipidus, thyroid disease (hyper or hypo), adrenal disorders, hypopituitarism (congenital or acquired).

  b. Non-organic (perhaps 75-90% of all FTT cases in some series; may be as low as 10-15% depending on population)

    1) Child may be "hyper-alert" with minimal vocalization vs. heightened response to strangers.

    2) Pale, loss of muscle mass.

    3) May have tonic immobility (flexed).

    4) History of feeding problem; difficult temperament; being unplanned/unwanted, the youngest; parental history of abuse, FTT, depression; lack of involved father; distant/overwrought mother; lack of social supports, poor preventive health care (delinquent immunizations); history of multiple medical providers.

    5) If hospitalized, 2/3 improve away from home; however, may require 3-4 <u>weeks</u>!

    6) Usually decreased growth hormone and iron parameters, delayed bone age.

5. Evaluation

  a. Immediate hospitalization advisable if abuse/neglect suspected, child is ill, or treatable organic disease is present. Probably should hospitalize any child with FTT within 1-2 mo of growth deceleration.

  b. Investigate organic and non-organic etiologies simultaneously (preferably with supportive, multidisciplinary approach).

  c. Complete history/physical/developmental assessment.

  d. Initial laboratory tests - cbc with diff, serum electrolytes, BUN, creatinine, and glucose; U/A and culture; stool exam for reducing substances and fat; tine; $\pm$ CXR.

  e. Other tests as dictated by history, PE: radiographic assessment of GI tract, ECG, bone age (unreliable if very young), sweat test, radiographic assessment of GU tract. The less evident an organic history is at presentation, the less likely laboratory tests are to find one.

  One study examined 185 children with FTT who received 2607 laboratory tests; only 10 (0.4%) established diagnosis and only 26 (1.0%) supported diagnosis.

  f. Calorie count/observed feeding trial.

6. Treatment is directed toward underlying cause. Children with non-organic FTT and their parents merit family counseling/psychotherapy. Unfortunately only 33% will be normal at follow-up 5-10 years later, and 50% will be delayed or experience learning/personal problems.

C. Hypertension

1. The measurement of BP is a necessary part of the PE.

  a. In neonates, infants, and toddlers, BP may be more easily measured by Doppler than by auscultation.

  b. In older children and adolescents, the manual method is convenient.

    1) The child is seated with his arm at heart level.

    2) The blood pressure cuff is wrapped around the upper arm (the bladder should encircle the arm and cover 2/3 of its length) and is inflated to about 2 mm Hg above the point at which the radial pulse disappears.

    3) Observing the manometer (anaeroid or mercury), the cuff is deflated at a rate of 2mm/second.

    4) Auscultation over the brachial artery reveals the onset of an audible tapping sound (systolic pressure, Korotkoff I sound); further

deflation and auscultation reveals a muffled sound (Korotkoff IV) and finally, its disappearance (Korotkoff V).

5) Because there is debate as to which sound (IV or V) truly represents diastole, both are recorded (e.g., 110/70/64).

6) Since some children have heart sounds audible throughout the cuff's deflation, the Korotkoff IV sound has been used in age and sex-appropriate BP standards.

2. Inaccurate BP measurements occur when the cuff size is incorrect (especially too small), the patient is moving, crying, or upset, or the equipment is not calibrated correctly. Observer bias also occurs.

3. When a healthy child has either a systolic or diastolic pressure between the 90th and 95th percentiles for age and sex, he is said to have high normal BP. If a child's systolic and/or diastolic pressures equal or exceed the 95%ile on three separate occasions, he has persistently elevated blood pressure (hypertension).

4. Causes of Hypertension

a. Renal (acute glomerulonephritis; hemolytic uremic syndrome; nephrosis; lupus; trauma; renal arterial disease (trauma, congenital defects, acquired disease); obstructive uropathy (posterior urethral valves, ureteroceles, bladder diverticuli, ureterovesicular/ureteropelvic obstruction); congenital disorders (polycystic renal disease, dysplasia, hypoplasia); tumors, lead nephropathy; mercury poisoning; radiation nephritis; S/P GU surgery/renal transplant/ renal rejection; end-stage-renal disease).

b. Vascular (renal vessel anomalies, thrombosis, or stenosis; aortitis, aortic coarctation either in the thoracic or abdominal areas).

c. Endocrine (primary hyperparathyroidism, primary hyperthyroidism, pheochromocytoma, neuroblastoma, Cushing's syndrome, adreno-

genital syndrome, 11-hydroxylase and 17-hydroxylase deficiencies, primary aldosteronism).
  d. Miscellaneous (collagen-vascular disease, poliomyelitis; Guillain-Barré syndrome; dysautonomia; porphyria; hypercalcemia; Stevens-Johnson syndrome; therapy with sympathomimetics, steroids, or oral contraceptives; amphetamine abuse; burns; malignancies; SBE; and increased intracranial pressure).
  e. Primary hypertension occurs in the absence of conditions known to elevate blood pressure. Both genetics and environment (low socioeconomic status, high salt intake) may play a role in its genesis. Many children are asymptomatic; symptoms, when present, include frontal headaches, fatigue, epistaxis, and nervousness. Obesity is present in 50% of the children.
5. When a child presents with a persistently elevated BP, important historical information includes
  a. The child's birth history.
  b. Presence of chronic conditions/chronic or recurrent symptoms (headache, epistaxis).
  c. Use of chronic medications.
  d. Growth patterns.
  e. Urinary tract infections or disorders.
  f. Diet history.
  g. Family history of hypertension or its complications (renal disease, myocardial infarction, stroke).
6. The PE must be complete since many causes of secondary hypertension have characteristic physical findings. Special emphasis is placed on the BP measured in both arms and one leg to R/O coarctation, and the right arm in supine, sitting, and standing positions. A fundoscopic exam (if abnormal, indicates hypertension has been present >1 year) and complete cardiac exam are mandatory.
7. Laboratory tests are dictated by the history and physical findings. A routine U/A, serum creati-

nine, BUN, uric acid, and cbc are useful screens. If the patient is obese, a fasting cholesterol (and its fractions) and high- and low-density lipoproteins are also useful. If the patient is a candidate for diuretics, serum electrolytes should be obtained. In any child for whom drug therapy is considered, a baseline echocardiogram is in order.

8. Management
   a. Treat the underlying condition if the hypertension is of the secondary type. However, a diuretic (see b6) and/or beta blocker (see b7) may still be necessary.
   b. Primary hypertension
      1) Weight loss to achieve ideal weight.
      2) Proper exercise.
      3) Limit salt intake.
      4) Avoid medications with sympathomimetics.
      5) Maintain positive attitude and patience with therapy.
      6) If #1-5 are unsuccessful, a thiazide diuretic may be useful (hydrochlorothiazide 1 mg/kg with a maximum of 2 mg/kg (200 mg) per day); potassium supplementation might be necessary.
      7) If the diuretic doesn't achieve BP control after 6-12 wk (and the diastolic pressure is 90-100 mm Hg in older children), one can add propranolol (a beta blocker) at an initial dose of 1 mg/kg/d or methyldopa (acts centrally on vasomotor centers and peripherally to decrease arteriolar resistance) at an initial dose of 5-10 mg/kg/d (max 65 mg/kg/d). Propanolol is contraindicated if the heart rate < 60/ min or if the patient has diabetes, asthma, heart disease, or ulcer disease.
      8) If a diuretic plus propranolol/methyldopa do not achieve good BP control, hydralazine (vasodilates peripheral arterioles by relaxing smooth muscles) is added at an initial dose of

1 mg/kg/d (max 5 mg/kg or 200 mg). Follow antinuclear antibodies since hydralazine has been reported to induce lupus.

9) Infants whose hypertension is refractory to other agents might be treated with captopril (see Hypertension ref. #7).

10) A hypertensive crisis (abrupt marked elevation in BP) can occur in renal disease, hemolytic-uremic syndrome, pheochromocytoma, renin-secreting tumors, and severe CNS pathology. Symptoms include headaches, diplopia, seizures, CHF, facial palsy, edema, and hypertensive retinopathy. Therapy varies by etiology.

   a) Acute glomerulonephritis: furosemide (1-2 mg/kg IV over minutes) plus hydralazine (0.15-0.2 mg/kg IV or IM over minutes) or diazoxide (1.5-5 mg/kg IV rapid bolus).

   b) Hemolytic-Uremic syndrome: furosemide and diazoxide (as above); may require peritoneal dialysis.

   c) Renal artery disease: multiple diazoxide doses or nitroprusside drip (1 µg/kg/m IV).

   d) End-stage renal disease: diazoxide (as above) or nitroprusside drip (as above).

   e) Pheochromocytoma: diazoxide (as above) or nitroprusside drip (as above) prior to surgery.

D. Joint Pain and Joint Swelling

1. Arthritis vs. Arthralgia
   a. Arthritis - swelling of a joint or limitation of motion accompanied by heat, pain, and tenderness.
   b. Arthralgia - subjective complaint of joint pain or tenderness without swelling or limitation of motion.

     c. Joint Swelling can occur secondary to:
       1) Periarticular soft-tissue swelling (angioneu-
         rotic edema, tenosynovitis),
       2) Thickened synovium (JRA),
       3) Joint effusion (septic arthritis, acute rheumat-
         ic fever, JRA, trauma),
       4) Bony enlargement (traumatic arthritis).
2. General

  Joint complaints are common in children. In most cases the problem is transient and is the result of trauma or strenuous activity. The patient needs to be evaluated carefully for evidence of tendonitis, myositis, myalgia, muscular or ligamentous strain. Pain and loss of motion can result from changes at musculoskeletal sites other than joints. Bone, muscle, nerve, and referred pain can all be confused with arthritis.

3. Evaluation
    a. History

      Which joints are involved? Characteristics: large joints, small joints, monarticular, polyarticular, symmetric, migratory, duration? Systemic manifestations: fever, rash, weight loss, stool abnormalities? Response to anti-inflammatories? Family history? Recent trauma, new activities, immunizations, exposure to infections (hepatitis, rubella, gonorrhea, mononucleosis?).

    b. Physical Exam

      Should be complete but focus on bone, joint, muscle, and nerve status. Useful findings include rash (JRA, Henoch-Schönlein purpura (HSP) serum sickness, gonococcal infection, Lyme disease, Kawasaki disease, inflammatory conditions), hepatosplenomegaly, lymphadenopathy, eye changes on slit-lamp exam, and a positive joint exam. Look for evidence of hypermobility (see Joint Pain/Swelling ref. 2).

    c. Laboratory Studies

      These should be based on the findings of the

history and physical examination.

1) CBC: leukocytosis favors infectious or inflammatory etiology.

2) ESR, CRP elevation favors an infectious or inflammatory etiology. An elevated ESR is <u>not</u> usually seen in traumatic, mechanical, orthopedic problems.

3) ANA, rheumatoid factor: helpful if positive, but not very sensitive tests.

4) Synovial fluid exam and culture, blood, throat, and stool cultures, mono test, viral titers (EBV) are all helpful in patients with suspected infection.

In patients with acute monarticular arthritis, an elevated ESR or CRP, temp >38.5 and leukocytosis are independent predictors for the diagnosis of septic arthritis.

In a patient whose symptoms exceed two weeks, a low CRP, absence of fever, and elevated IgG are independent predictors for the diagnosis of JRA.

5) Bone marrow aspiration: in patient with suspected malignancy.

6) Urinalysis: Henoch-Schönlein purpura.

d. Imaging

1) Radiography is indicated in patients with suspected orthopedic problems, i.e., trauma, Legg-Calvé-Perthes disease, slipped capital femoral epiphysis. Also for osteoid osteoma and malignancy.

2) Radionuclide joint and bone scans may be useful, i.e., malignancy, diskitis, osteoid osteoma, toddler's fracture, Legg-Calvé-Perthes. Bone scintigraphy is useful with occult bone and periosteal injuries (child abuse, sports injuries) and <u>may</u> differentiate among septic arthrtis, cellulitis, and osteomyelitis.

3) Ultrasonography of the hip is useful for joint effusion (transient synovitis) and thickened synovium.

4) CT may localize a foreign body in a patient with monarticular arthritis.

e. Arthroscopy
Useful for evaluation of traumatic/mechanical joint problems.

4. Differential Diagnosis

a. Trauma and Orthopedic Conditions
1) Child abuse
2) Femoral neck anteversion
3) Legg-Calvé-Perthes
4) Osgood-Schlatter
5) Osteochondritis dissecans
6) Osteoid osteoma
7) Slipped capital femoral epiphysis
8) Sports injuries
9) Subluxation/chondromalacia of the patella (patella-femoral pain syndrome)

b. Inflammatory
1) Acute rheumatic fever
2) Allergic reactions/serum sickness
3) Connective tissue disorders, i.e., systemic lupus erythematosis (SLE)
4) Inflammatory bowel disease
5) Juvenile rheumatoid arthritis
6) Psoriatic arthritis
7) Vasculitis: HSP, Kawasaki disease, periarteritis

c. Infections and Post-Infectious
1) Antecedent enterobacterial infections (<u>Salmonella, Shigella, Yersinia</u>)
2) Gonococcal
3) Lyme disease
4) <u>Mycoplasma</u>
5) Osteomyelitis
6) Periarticular cellulitis
7) Septic arthritis
8) Viral (hepatitis, mononucleosis, rubella)

d. Miscellaneous
1) Foreign body synovitis/arthritis

       2) Hypermobility syndromes
       3) Inflammatory bowel disease
       4) Malignancy
       5) Neuropathic arthropathy
       6) Psychogenic
       7) Sickle cell disease
       8) Transient synovitis of the hip
    e. Diagnostic Tips
       1) Fever and ESR are the most useful screening parameters. An elevation of either suggests an inflammatory or infectious origin.
       2) Absence of fever and a normal ESR are <u>strongly</u> against an inflammatory or infectious etiology, but may be seen in pauciarticular JRA.
       3) In monarticular disease, a positive joint exam in association with fever and/or an elevated ESR suggests septic arthritis or osteomyelitis.
       4) A positive joint exam <u>not</u> associated with fever or an elevated ESR suggests an orthopedic problem, but may also occur with JRA, SLE and psoriatic arthritis.
       5) Rash is predictive of inflammatory disorders.
5. Specific Disorders
    a. Gonococcal Arthritis
      There are two forms; GU infection is usually asymptomatic with both.
       1) Involvement of multiple large (knees, wrists, and ankles) and small joints, often in association with fever, chills, and skin lesions. Blood culture may be positive.
       2) Monarticular arthritis with minimal systemic signs and symptoms. Blood culture is negative but organisms may be recovered from a joint effusion as well as from skin lesions. May present as repeated episodes of tenosyovitis coincident with menses.
    b. Hypermobility Syndrome
      May occur with a number of syndromes or as a

distinct clinical entity. The patient usually presents with recurrent episodes of self-limited arthralgias involving multiple joints along with evidence of hypermobility. Episodes may last for several days to several weeks.

c. Juvenile Rheumatoid Arthritis (JRA)

Think of this diagnosis in patient with arthritis lasting more than 6 weeks in at least one joint, after exclusion of other possibilities.

May present in one of three forms:

1) Systemic: Multiple joints and prominent constitutional symptoms (rash, spiking fevers); <25% of patients.

2) Polyarticular: >4 joints; often symmetric and frequently involving the hands; minor systemic manifestations.

3) Pauciarticular: < 4 joints; rarely systemic involvement - young girls (<4 yr) with pauciarticular disease and + ANA are at high risk for uveitis.

Conditions often confused with JRA include soft tissue pain due to myalgia, malignancy, hypermobility syndromes, infectious arthritis, "growing pains," and psychogenic pain. Misdiagnosis is especially common in patients with monarticular disease.

ANA and rheumatoid factor screens are helpful if positive, but are not very sensitive.

d. Lyme Disease

1) Caused by spirochete and transmitted by tick.

2) Following the tick bite, 50% of patients develop characteristic skin lesion, erythema chronicum migrans. Starts as an erythematous papule or macule that develops into an expanding erythematous annular lesion with central clearing. It may reach a diameter of 20-60 cm. Common on thigh, groin, and axilla; 50% have multiple lesions.

3) Associated manifestations include malaise, fever, headache and musculoskeletal pains.

4) Weeks to months following rash, patient may develop neurologic manifestations (meningoencephalitis, chorea, facial palsy, myelitis), cardiac complications (A-V conduction defects) or arthritis.

5) Arthritis presents abruptly with swelling, pain, and redness and is usually monarticular. It occurs in large joints such as the knee, but may affect the smaller joints of the hands and feet. Episodes may last for weeks to months and may recur over several years.

6) Serology (IFA and Elisa) can be used for laboratory confirmation.

7) Early treatment with tetracycline or penicillin may attenuate or prevent arthritis and other late complications. Active joint disease is treated with anti-inflammatory agents and a prolonged course of penicillin.

8) There is often severe joint pain out of proportion to the degree of arthritis. Episodes may be transient, recurrent, or persistent, and there may be intermittent fevers.

e. Malignancies

Patient may present with localized or diffuse bone pain or "arthritis" as an early sign of unrecognized malignancy (leukemia, neuroblastoma). There may be true arthritis secondary to bony, capsular, or periosteal lesions. Extreme joint pain or refusal to walk 2° to joint pain should always raise the suspicion of malignancy.

Radiographs, radionuclide scans, and bone marrow aspirates are eventually diagnostic but may not become positive for many months.

f. Mechanical Problems

Complaints are often chronic and diagnosis suggested by history. In the absence of fever and an elevated ESR, a positive joint exam suggests an orthopedic disorder. Radiography may be helpful.

g. Septic Arthritis

1) In a patient with acute monarticular arthritis, an elevated ESR or CRP, temp >38.5°C and leukocytosis are highly suggestive of septic arthritis. Cultures of blood and joint fluid are mandatory.

2) The knee, hip, and ankle are the most commonly affected joints.

3) Over age 5 years, usually associated with trauma or skin infection (S. aureus); under age 5 years, usually associated with URI symptoms (H. influenzae type B).

4) Bone scintigraphy can occasionally be useful in differentiating septic arthritis from osteomyelitis and periarticular cellulitis.

h. Transient Synovitis of the Hip

1) Differential diagnosis of hip pain includes Legg-Calvé-Perthes (aseptic necrosis), infection, psoas abscess, arthritis, slipped capital femoral epiphysis, and transient synovitis.

2) Transient synovitis is the most probable diagnosis in a child <10 years with an acute limp and hip pain, often following a URI or trauma. There may be decreased range of motion and referred knee pain.

3) The diagnosis is supported by the presence of joint effusion on ultrasound, absence of fever, and a low CRP or ESR.

E. Mucocutaneous Lymph Node Syndrome (Kawasaki)

1. Mucocutaneous lymph node syndrome (MLNS) is an acute exanthematous illness of childhood. Patients are usually <5 years (peak incidence 6-24

months) with a male-to-female ratio of 1.5:1. There is a 1-2% mortality rate in the subacute or early convalescent stage, usually from cardiovascular complications.

2. MLNS is triphasic:
   a. Acute febrile stage (days 1-4) (stars indicate diagnostic criteria)
      *1) Fever - Intermittent, spiking (> 40°C) only temporarily responsive to antipyretics; must be present at least 5 d before a diagnosis of MLNS is considered.
      *2) Conjunctival injection - occur within 2-3 d of fever's onset; bilateral, non-purulent, especially marked in bulbar conjunctivae.
      *3) Oral mucosal findings - occur within 1-3 d of fever's onset; reddened fissured lips, reddened oropharynx, and "strawberry" tongue.
      *4) Rash - occurs with onset of fever; takes several forms (erythematous, irregular plaques that are partially confluent; morbilliform eruption; scarlatiniform; urticarial); rash occurs principally on face and trunk; is <u>never</u> vesicular, bullous, petechial, purpuric, or crusting.
      *5) Extremity changes - occur within several days of fever's onset; palms and soles develop a red edema that is indurative and tender; skin of dorsum of hands and feet appears shiny and stretched.
      *6) Lymphadenopathy - usually not generalized, but frequently a solitary cervical node ($\geq$ 1.5 cm in diameter) that is rarely warm, tender, or fluctuant.
      7) Behavioral changes - irritability, lethargy; mood lability.
      8) Abdominal pain, diarrhea, liver inflammation, anorexia.
      9) GU signs and symptoms (sterile pyuria, urethritis, hematuria).

10) Joint involvement (late in first stage).

11) Cardiovascular involvement (perivasculitis and microvasculitis of coronary arteries, aorta microvasculitis, pancarditis); usually not clinically apparent.

12) Significant laboratory findings: elevated ESR and CRP; pyuria; elevated (>20,000) wbc with left shift; thrombocytosis (end of this stage); negative cultures.

b. Subacute stage (days 15-25): The fever, rash and lymphadenopathy subside. Conjunctivae may still be red; oral mucosal changes are still present. Peripheral extremities begin to desquamate starting periungually and moving proximally between days 10 and 20; skin on other parts of the body may also desquamate. Anorexia and mood changes are still present.

1) Joint involvement - arthralgias/arthritis in large joints (knees, hips, elbows); effusion(s) may be present.

2) Cardiac disease - improving pancarditis; coronary arteries demonstrate persistent panvasculitis and may demonstrate areas of thrombosis. Coronary artery aneurysms develop in 20% of MLNS patients. Clinically, there may be tachycardia, a gallop, muffled heart sounds, minor ECG changes (prolonged PR interval, ST/T wave changes); more severely ill children may have cardiomyopathy with CHF, pericardial effusion, and mitral valve insufficiency. Sudden death may occur due to aneurysm rupture or coronary artery occlusion.

3) Significant laboratory findings (tests abnormal in first stage are usually still abnormal; thrombocytosis - usually 600,000-1,000,000; mild anemia; and elevated AST, CPK and LDH if myocarditis).

c. Convalescent stage (days 26-60): Eyes, oral

mucosa, extremities, mood, joint symptoms, and appetite are all improving or normal. Early in this stage, coronary artery inflammation is still present; sudden death is still a threat. By the end of this stage, the arteries have developed scars in their walls and recanalization of their lumens.

Most abnormal laboratory values have normalized by the end of this stage.

3. Differential diagnosis in early stage: rash may be confused with that caused by measles, Group A <u>Streptococcus</u>, Epstein-Barr virus, leptospirosis, drug eruption, or erythema multiforme.

4. Risk factors have been identified to detect the children most likely to develop coronary aneurysms or thrombosis. Children with ≤ 5 factors generally do well; those with >9 are at high risk.
   a. Male sex
   b. Age <1 year
   c. Duration of initial fever >15 d
   d. Recrudescent rash
   e. WBC >30,000
   f. Westergren sedimentation rate >100
   g. Presence of cardiomegaly
   h. Presence of arrhythmias
   i. Recrudescent fever
   j. Evidence of myocardial infarction
   k. Prolonged QR interval
   l. Hemoglobin <10
   m. Elevated ESR >5 wk

5. Management
   a. Acute stage
      1) Appropriate work-up to R/O sepsis, meningitis (if indicated), treatable infections.
      2) Baseline cbc, ESR, CRP, liver/cardiac enzymes, chest film, ECG.
      3) May need to hospitalize for observation or intravenous fluids; if not hospitalized, child needs to be seen 2-4 times/week.

4) Abnormal lab results should be checked <u>at least weekly</u> (and in many cases twice/week).

5) If an outpatient develops cardiac symptoms or abnormalities, he should be immediately hospitalized.

6) Aspirin should be given (80-100 mg/kg/d) to maintain a serum salicylate level of 20 mg/dl.

7) Immune globulin-400 mg/kg/day IV x 3 days: should be given as soon as possible after diagnosis.

8) Do not use steroids! (increase platelet counts and associated with higher incidence of coronary aneurysms).

9) Echocardiogram at end of first stage.

b. Subacute stage

1) After defervescence, the aspirin dose may be halved (monitor serum salicylate levels); however, children with coronary artery abnormalities should continue on high-dose aspirin.

2) Cardiac exam, cbc, ESR, platelet count, and ECG should be serially monitored.

3) Repeat echocardiogram (compare with initial one).

4) Supportive therapy.

5) If CHF, appropriate therapy.

6) Coronary angiogram if child presents with infarction or coronary vessel damage.

c. Convalescent stage

1) Children with normal echos should have a repeat study when platelet counts normalize (2-3 mo). If no abnormalities are found, aspirin therapy is stopped, and the child is seen q 1-3 mo for follow-up.

2) Children with evidence of aneurysms should have serial echos to assess aneurysm change. A repeat angiogram is indicated in a year.

3) Children with increasing cardiac symptoms or vessel involvement may require bypass surgery.

F. Lymphadenopathy

1. General Guidelines

   In evaluation of child with lymphadenopathy the following points can be helpful in differential diagnosis.

2. Size

   Nodes under 3mm in diameter are normal. Up to age 12, cervical and inguinal nodes up to 1 cm and epitrochlear nodes up to 0.5 cm may be normal. Nodes > 2 cm are suspicious of granulomatous disease or tumor.

3. Location

   a. Hodgkin's - supraclavicular and lower neck.

   b. Cat-scratch-preauricular, axillary, inguinal, epitrochlear.

   c. Reactive hyperplasia - inguinal, submental, posterior cervical.

   d. Atypical mycobacterial - upper cervical, submandibular, preauricular.

   N.B. Generalized adenopathy is usually due to generalized disease.

4. Duration

   Not that helpful in suggesting diagnosis. If node increases after 2 week F/U <u>or</u> has not decreased after 4-6 week F/U, biopsy is indicated.

5. Consistency

   a. Matted or fixed nodes - neoplasm or granulomatous disease.

   b. Tender nodes with overlying erythema - bacterial adenitis.

   The <u>more tender</u> the node, the <u>less ominous</u> the diagnosis.

6. Age

   a. < 4 yr - reactive hyperplasia, atypical mycobacterium.

    b. > 8 yr - reactive hyperplasia, cat-scratch, Hodgkin's (especially in teengers).

7. Associated Signs and Symptoms
Liver/spleen enlargement, prolonged fever, weight loss suggestive of serious systemic illness (malignancy).

8. History
    a. Exposure to TB, cats? Medication history (i.e., Dilantin).
    b. The most common cause of cervical adenopathy in children is bacterial/viral infection in the ENT area.
    c. Generalized adenopathy (2 or more non-contiguous lymph node groups) is usually due to reactive hyperplasia. This is by far the most common diagnosis in children who come to biopsy.
    d. If patient is febrile >1 week, R/O mononucleosis, CMV, toxoplasmosis, Kawasawki.

9. Workup includes history, PE, cbc, ESR, PPD, mono test, TC, viral titers, CXR. Role of needle aspiration is controversial; most significant treatable conditions are best diagnosed by biopsy.

10. Timing of lymph node biopsy.
In general indications for biopsy include:
    a. Unexplained fever and weight loss,
    b. Fixation of node to overlying skin or underlying tissue,
    c. Supraclavicular location,
    d. Abnormal CXR (strongest predictor of serious disease)
    e. Increase in size of node after several weeks of observation.

11. The following scoring system may be useful in adolescents:

Abnormal CXR	5 points
Lymph node > 2 cm	3 points
ENT symptoms	-3 points
Constant	-2 points

a. If score is >0 - biopsy will probably lead to treatment.

b. If score is <0 - watch, will probably not alter treatment.

c. The greater the score, the more likely it is to be correct.

d. Even after biopsy, a specific etiology may be established in only 40% of children. The most common histologic diagnoses are: reactive hyperplasia, neoplastic disease, granulomatous disease.

N.B. Approximately 20% of children who initially have a non-diagnostic biopsy will eventually develop a specific pathologic process - patients need close F/U.

C. Specific Causes of Lymphadenopathy

1. Atypical Mycobacterium
   a. Children 1-6 yr.
   b. Unilateral matted, fixed nodes without tenderness.
   c. CXR negative; PPD negative or weakly positive.
   d. Diagnosis - excisional biopsy; needle aspiration or I + D may lead to chronic draining sinus tract.
   e. Treatment - total excision; anti-TB drugs are ineffective.

2. Lymphoma
   a. > 8 yr; usually teenagers.
   b. Rubbery, matted or fixed, non-tender nodes.
   c. Supraclavicular and lower cervical location.

    d. Liver/spleen enlargement, fever, weight loss, anemia, abnormal CXR-mediastinal or hilar adenopathy.

    e. Diagnosis - biopsy.

  3. Cat-Scratch Disease

    a. > 8 yr.

    b. Single or multiple nodes; usually tender; suppuration in 15%.

    c. Parotid, preauricular, axillary, epitrochlear, inguinal.

    d. May be malaise, fatigue, low-grade fever; history of cat exposure; may be crusted papule, vesiculo-pustule or ulcer distal to node.

    e. Diagnosis is by clinical picture; characteristic histologic picture; cat-scratch skin test is helpful but antigen may be hard to obtain.

    f. Treatment - none.

  4. Viral

    a. Any age.

    b. Discrete, mobile, soft consistency; no redness or warmth; may be tender.

    c. Upper anterior cervical, posterior cervical, generalized.

    d. Associated fever, malaise, URI syptoms; liver/spleen enlargement.

    e. Diagnosis - serologic studies.

    N.B. CMV and toxoplasmosis may be indistinguishable from EBV infection.

G. Myositis

Excruciating pain in the calf muscles in association with signs and symptoms of a viral illness is seen in children secondary to Asian influenza B infection. The muscles are tender to palpation and children will often refuse to bear weight or walk. It usually resolves in several days. Treatment consists of acetaminophen and warm baths. CPK may be extremely elevated. Rarely may be associated with widespread muscle necrosis with myoglobinuria and acute tubular necrosis.

H. Reye's Syndrome

1. S/SX:
   a. Picture of acute toxic encephalopathy in association with hepatic dysfunction. Usual presentation is nausea and vomiting during recovery from viral illness (varicella, influenza) followed by irritability or combative behavior, confusion, decreased responsiveness, and lethargy. Stupor, loss of DTRs, decerebrate posture, convulsions, and coma are seen later in the course. <u>No</u> focal neurologic signs. Liver may be moderately enlarged.
   b. <u>Infants</u> may present with sudden onset of respiratory distress (tachypnea, apneic episodes) followed by seizures and coma +/- vomiting. Hypoglycemia usually prominent.
2. Lab abnormalities
   a. ↑ Transaminases, ammonia, prothrombin time, creatinine phosphokinase, organic and amino acids.
   b. Bilirubin usually normal; CSF is normal.
   c. Hypoglycemia primarily in children <4 yr.
   d. EEG - generalized slow-wave abnormalities.
3. Case Definition (CDC)
   a. Acute non-inflammatory encephalopathy with one of the following:
      1) Fatty metamorphosis of the liver.
      2) AST, ALT or serum ammonia >3x normal.
   b. CSF (if obtained) <8 WBC.
   c. No other more reasonable explanation for the neurologic or hepatic abnormalities.
      N.B. Acute deterioration may be seen following LP. May be best to defer until ICP can be measured. CT may be helpful. If LP must be done, use small gauge needle and remove as little CSF as possible.

4. Differential Dx:
   a. Urea cycle disorders.
   b. Encephalitis, meningitis, septicemia.
   c. Toxins - salicylate poisoning, valproic acid, iso-propyl alcohol.
   d. Acute hepatitis with coma.
   e. Carnitine deficiency.
   f. Organic acidurias.
5. Staging
   a. 0 - no neurologic signs.
   b. I - subtle CNS changes - confusion, listless, apathy; normal posture, pain response, and pupillary reactions.
   c. II - delirious, restlessness, irritability, disorientation, combativeness, normal posture, sluggish pupils, conjugate deviation of the eyes.
   d. III - deep coma, decorticate posturing, sluggish pupils, conjugate deviation of the eyes.
   e. IV - coma, decerebrate posture, sluggish pupils, spinal state - flaccid, areflexia, apnea, nonreactive pupils, absent doll's eyes.
   All patients with <u>presumptive</u> Reye's syndrome, regardless of stage, should promptly be transferred to intensive care unit capable of caring for such patients.

I. Stinging Insect Reactions (Bees, Wasps, Hornets)

1. Small local reaction
   a. Small urticarial lesions with erythema and pruritus; last several hours.
   b. Treatment: none.
2. Large local reactions
   a. Swelling at sting site of >5 cm; may involve entire extremity and last as long as one week.
   b. Treatment: ice; po antihistamine; analgesic; short course of po prednisone may be used but efficacy not documented.
3. Generalized urticaria, erythema, pruritus, and angioedema

       a. Treatment: SQ epinephrine 1:1000 - 0.01 cc/kg up to 0.3 cc: may repeat in 15 minutes.
       b. Skin testing and immunotherapy not indicated.
       c. Patient should have epinephrine kit available for self-injection (Epi-Pen).
       d. Careful instructions about insect avoidance.
    4. Life-Threatening reactions
       a. Laryngeal edema, bronchospasm, hypotension
       b. Treatment: SQ epinephrine 1:1000 - 0.01 cc/kg up to 0.3 cc, oxygen, volume expanders, pressor agents, airway support.
       c. Steroids not generally effective - delayed onset of action.
       d. Patient should be referred to allergist for skin-testing and possible venom immunotherapy.
       e. Patient should always carry epinephrine self-injector (Epi-Pen).
       N.B. In general, stinging insect reactions are rarely fatal in children and tendency to severe reactions tends to diminish with time.

J. Substance Abuse

1. Recognizing the Adolescent Substance Abuser

       a. 60-70% of teenagers "experiment" with various drugs at some time; 10-15% have problems related to the use of alcohol and other drugs; 1-5% are chemically dependent.
       b. Substance abuse is usually underidentified by health professionals. Adolescents rarely present with chemical dependency as a primary or secondary complaint. Clinical signs and symptoms of dependence are unusual in the adolescent drug abuser. Signs and symptoms of withdrawal are unusual. However, acute overdoses and adverse reactions are a major problem.
       c. Risk factors for substance abuse
          1) Family history of alcoholism and other drug use.
          2) History of verbal, physical, or sexual abuse.

3) Antisocial behavior (conduct disorders); rebeliousness.
4) Academic underachievement.
5) Developmental disabilities.
6) Poor self-esteem; alienation.
7) Friends who use drugs.
8) Early first use of drugs.
   Classic picture includes personality change, poor family interactions, deteriorating school performance, and withdrawal from positive environmental factors (church, sports, extra-curricular activities).

d. Think of substance abuse in adolescent who:
   1) Shows unexplained or out-of-the ordinary behavior, e.g., depression, emotional change.
   2) Presents with fatigue, non-specific symptoms, or psychosomatic complaints.
   3) Presents with injuries related to falls, fighting, motor vehicle accidents, or near-drowning.
   4) Attempts suicide - 1/2 to 2/3 of young suicides have a history of substance abuse (usually multiple drugs over many yrs).

2. General approach to patient with acute drug abuse reaction

   a. Gastric decontamination
      1) Induce emesis - syrup of ipecac if alert or gastric lavage after intubation.
      2) Activated charcoal.
      3) Cathartic.
   b. Establish an airway and support ventilation.
   c. Start IV and support cardiac output.
   d. If patient is obtunded, give IV or IM naloxone 0.4-2 mg.
   e. Initial Evaluation
      1) Talk to friends, parents, associates, paramedics. Was the usage recreational, episodic, experimental or habitual? Was the overuse

intentional or accidental?

2) Complete PE; check for associated trauma; establish neurologic flow sheet and Glasgow coma scale.

3) Check patient's clothing for clues to the ingested substance; identify any recovered substances; utilize local poison control center.

f. Obtain urine and blood for toxicology screens (important to know what the screen does and does not pick up).

g. Depending on initial workup, obtain: ABGs, electrolytes, blood glucose, BUN, creatinine, LFTs, serum ketones, urinalysis.

h. Reassurance and psychological support; restraint and force should be avoided if at all possible.

3. Specific acute drug abuse reactions
   a. Alcohol
      1) Clinical manifestations
         (a) Mental Status: aggressive, belligerent behavior, impaired mentation, sleepiness, slurred speech.
         (b) Physical exam: ataxia, constricted pupils (dilated after extreme intoxication), hypotension, hypothermia; respiratory depression, tachycardia; (look for signs of associated trauma, aspiration).
         (c) Withdrawal syndrome: anxiety, insomnia, irritability. Severe withdrawal (convulsions, delirium, hallucinations) is rarely seen in adolescents.
      2) Treatment: supportive care and correction of metabolic abnormalities (hypoglycemia, acidosis).
   b. Anticholinergics
      Atropine, belladonna, benztropine, henbane, jimson weed seed, procyclidine, propantheline bromide, scopolamine, trihexyphenidyl

1) Clinical Manifestations
   (a) Mental Status: amnesia, body image alteration, clouded sensorium, coma, confusion, convulsions, disorientation, drowsiness, restlessness, violent behavior, visual hallucinations.
   (b) Physical exam: dilated pupils, dry skin, flushed, hyperthermia, tachycardia, decreased bowel sound, urinary retention.
   (c) Withdrawal syndrome: gastrointestinal and musculoskeletal symptoms.
2) Treatment: supportive care. Physostigmine (which has serious adverse effects) should be reserved for treatment of life-threatening manifestations including coma, respiratory depression, severe hypertension, and uncontrollable convulsions.

c. Cannabis Group
   Marijuana, hashish, THC, hash oil, <u>Sinsemilla (marijuana)</u>
   1) Clinical Manifestations
      (a) Mental Status: anxiety; anorexia, then increased appetite; confusion; depersonalization; dreamy, fantasy state; euphoria; excitement; hallucinations; panic reactions; paranoia; time-space distortions.
      (b) Physical exam: ataxia, dry hacking cough, injected conjunctiva, postural hypotension, tachycardia.
      (c) Withdrawal syndrome: anorexia, anxiety, depression, insomnia, irritability, nausea, restlessness. Acute withdrawal reactions are rare.
   2) Treatment: no specific treatment is indicated. Diazepam may be used for severe anxiety or panic reactions.

d. CNS Depressants (downers)
   Barbiturates, benzodiazepines, chloral hydrate, ethylchlorvynol, glutethimide, meprobamate,

methaqualone, methyprylon, paraldehyde.
1) Clinical Manifestations
   (a) Mental Status: coma, confusion, delirium, disorientation, drowsiness, slurred speech.
   (b) Physical exam: ataxia, convulsions (methaqualone), hyporeflexia, hypotension, hypothermia, hypotonia, nystagmus, pulmonary edema, respiratory depression.
   (c) Withdrawal syndrome: agitation, anxiety, arrhythmias, convulsions, delirium, disorientation, fever, hallucinations, hyperreflexia, hypertension, insomnia, irritabiltiy, sweating, tremors, weakness, cardiovascular collapse.
2) Treatment: supportive care, maintain airway and ventilation, support BP, forced diuresis, alkalinization of urine; hemodialysis may be indicated with high blood drug levels of long-acting agents.

N.B. Acute withdrawal can be life-threatening. The drug dosage may need to be tapered, or phenobarbital or pentobarbital substituted and the dosage gradually decreased.

e. CNS Stimulants (uppers)
   Amphetamine, amphetamine-like anti-obesity drugs, Bromo-DMA, caffeine, dextroamphetamine, diethyl propion, MDA, MDMA, methylphenidate, phenmetrazine, phenylpropanolamine.
   1) Clinical Manifestations
      (a) Mental Status: agitation, anxiety, decreased appetite, decreased sleep, delirium, hallucinations, hyperactivity, hyperacute or confused sensorium, impulsivity, paranoid ideation, restlessness.
      (b) Physical exam: arrythmias, blurred vision, coma, convulsions, dilated pupils, dry mouth, hyperreflexia, hypertension, hyperthermia, hyperventilation, stroke,

sweating, tachycardia, tremors.
- (c) Withdrawal syndrome: anxiety, chills, depression, exhaustion, muscular aches, sleep disturbances, tremors, voracious appetite.

2) Treatment: supportive care; "talk patient down;" chlorpromazine for aggressiveness, agitation, and hallucinations; diazepam for control of agitation and seizures; forced diuresis and acidification of urine. After patient has "crashed," a mild antidepressant (i.e., nortriptyline) can be given.

f. Cocaine
1) Clinical Manifestations
- (a) Mental status: (see CNS stimulants) agitation, hallucinations, panic, paranoid, psychosis, mood elevation, increased concentration.
- (b) Physical exam: arrhythmia, coma, convulsions, dilated pupils, hyperpnea, hyperreflexia, hypertension, hyperthermia, myocardial infarction, respiratory failure, sweating, stroke, tachycardia, epistaxis.
  Epiglottitis has been reported secondary to smoking cocaine.
- (c) Withdrawal syndrome: depression, irritability.

2) Treatment: support of ventilation; IV propranalol for cardiotoxicity; IV diazepam for seizures; cooling blanket for hyperthermia.

g. Hallucinogens
DMT; LSD; MDMA; Mescaline; morning glory seeds, nutmeg; psilocybin.
1) Clinical Manifestations
- (a) Mental Status: anxiety, confusion, convulsions/ depersonalization, depression, euphoria, hallucinations, illusions, inappropriate affect, panic, paranoia, synesthesias, time and visual distortions.

(b) Physical exam: dilated pupils, hyperreflexia, hypertension, hyperthermia, tachycardia, tremors.

(c) Withdrawal syndrome: none.

2) Treatment: supportive care, psychologic support ("talking down" in quiet area), mild tranquilizer for extreme anxiety, IM haloperidol for severe agitation, IV diazepam for sedation, cooling blanket for hyperthermia. <u>Avoid antipsychotic drugs</u>.

h. Opioids

Codeine, fentanyl, heroin, hydromorphine, meperidine, methadone, morphine, opium, pentazocine, propoxyphene, sufentanil.

1) Clinical Manifestations

(a) Mental Status: euphoria, stupor.

(b) Physical Exam: coma, constricted pupils, convulsions, hyporeflexia, hypotension, hypothermia, hypoventilation, pulmonary edema.

(c) Withdrawal syndrome: abdominal cramps, anxiety, diarrhea, dilated pupils, gooseflesh, lacrimation, muscle jerks, tachycardia, tremulousness, vomiting, yawning.

2) Treatment: IV or IM naloxone, 0.4-2 mg initially followed by continuous IV infusion of 2/3 of total initial dose q1h; positive end-expiratory pressure for pulmonary edema.

Withdrawal can be treated by giving po methadone 10 mg tid during first 24 h followed by lower doses.

i. Phencyclidine (PCP)

1) Clinical Manifestations

(a) Mental Status: amnesia; anxiety; coma; convulsions; excitement; hallucinations; hyperactivity; impulsive, self-destructive, or violent behavior; mutism; stupor; psychosis.

(b) Physical exam: ataxia, drooling, dysrythmia, flushing, hypertension, hyperthermia, hyporeflexia, myoclonus, nystagmus, open-eyed coma, tachycardia. Always evaluate patient carefully for signs of trauma.

(c) Withdrawal syndrome: none.

2) Treatment: psychological support; observation in a quiet area (do not "talk down"); IV diazepam for sedation and convulsions; haloperidol, 5 mg IM q 20 minutes until improved, for severe agitation; forced diuresis and acidifcation or urine; protect from harm; propranolol for dysrythmias. Admission for psychological evaluation is frequently required.

j. Volatile Substances

1) Aliphatic and aromatic hydrocarbons (gasoline, toluene, benzene, xylene); halogenated hydrocarbons (freons, halothane, trichlorethylene); aliphatic nitrites (amyl, m-butyl, and isobutyl nitrate); nitrous oxide.

2) Inhalants are frequently the first consciousness-altering substances used by children. They are popular because of rapid onset of action, quality and pattern of the "high," low cost, easy availability, convenient packaging, and the fact that possession is not illegal in most states.

3) Clinical Symptoms

(a) Mental status: confusion, convulsions, disorientation, dizziness, euphoria, hallucinations, headache, impulsive behavior, psychosis, somnolence; stupor.

(b) Physical exam: arrythmias, ataxia, coughing, drooling, hyporeflexia, hypotension, peripheral neuropathy, sneezing, tachycardia.

(c) Withdrawal syndrome: none.

N.B. Some volatiles may be associated with acute renal failures, DIC, hemolytic anemia, hypokalemia, methemoglobinemia, renal tubular acidosis.

(d) Treatment: supportive, maintenance of adequate ventilation.

4. Glossary of Drugs of Abuse

Abbots - Nembutal (pentobarbital) capsules, each marked with the manufacturer's name: "Abbott"

Acapulco Gold - very potent marijuana

Aimes (or Aymes, or Amys) - Amyl nitrite

All Star - Multiple-drug user

Angel Mist - PCP (phencyclidine)

Animal - LSD (lysergic acid diethylamide)

Baby - Marijuana. A small, irregular drug habit. As in a baby habit

Bad Seed - Peyote buttons

Bam - Amphetamine pill/capsules. Amphetamine prepared for injection

Barbs - Barbiturates, no specific brand name. Jagged edges of old hypodermic needles

Beans - Benzedrine (amphetamine)

Belly Habit - Opiate addiction

Benny's - Amphetamine

Benny Jag - To be high on amphetamines

Big C - Cocaine

Big Harry - Heroin

Black Cadillacs - Biphetamine (dextroamphetamine and amphetamine) 20 mg capsules

Black Dex - Biphetamine (dextroamphetamine and amphetamine) 20 mg capsules

Black Russian - Dark, very potent, hashish, possibly mixed with opium

Blanco - Heroin

Blotter - LSD

Blue Berkley - LSD, similar to "blotter," in which LSD drops are put on one-inch squares of blue paper and left to dry. This allows for easy transport of drug, and ingestion when paper is taken by mouth.

Blues - Barbiturates

Bombital/Bombito - Amphetamine or cocaine prepared for injection

Brown - Mexican heroin

Brown Slime - Nutmeg

Brown Mescaline - Brown powder, reported to contain mescaline

Brownstuff - Opium

Businessman's lunch - Dimethyltryptamine (DMT)

Busy Bee - PCP

Button - Mescaline

Candy - Cocaine, sometimes known as "nose candy," or any drug

Cartwheels - White, double-scored, amphetamine tablets, usually from illicit manufacturers

Chalk - Amphetamine tablets, usually from illicit manufacturers. These tablets have a white, gritty appearance, like chalk.

Channel - Vein used for injection

Chicago Green - Marijuana mixed with opium

Chiva - Heroin

Copilots - Amphetamine tablets/capsules

Cotton Habit - Irregular heroin habit

Courage Pills - Barbiturates

Crank - Amphetamine, usually from an illicit manufacturer

Cross - Amphetamine, usually from an illicit manufacturer, which is white, tablet form, and double scored.

Crossroads - See Cross

Crosstops - See Cross

Crystal - Amphetamine in powder form. PCP in solid form.

Dice - Methamphetamine, possibly Desoxyn

Dirt - Heroin

DOA - PCP

Dollies - Methadone

Dors and Fours - Doriden and Tylenol #4

Downers - Amytal (Amobarbital) capsules, Doriden (glutethimide)

Downs - Dalmane (flurazepam hydrochloride)

Drivers - Amphetamine, short for "truckdrivers," a term used to identify amphetamine

Dust - Cocaine, heroin, PCP, or morphine

Dusting - Mixing heroin and/or PCP with marijuana for smoking

Electric Kool-Aid - LSD mixed with punch

Elephant - PCP

Endurets - Preludin (phenmetrazine hydrochloride) prolonged-action tablets

F-40s - Seconal (secobarbital), 10 mg capsules, which are marked with the identification code "F-40"

F-66 - Tuinal (amobarbital sodium and secobarbital sodium), 200 mg capsule, which is marked with the identification code "F-66"

Fit - Equipment for injecting drugs

Fives - Amphetamine tablets, 5 mg each

Flea Powder - Highly diluted heroin

Flying Saucers - Morning glory seeds

Footballs - Amphetamine tablets in oval form. Dilaudid (hydromorphone) tablets

Fours - Tylenol (acetaminophen) with codeine #4 (60 mg of codeine per tablet)

Fuel - Marijuana sprayed or mixed with insecticides then smoked

Gin - Alcoholic beverage. Cocaine

Gold - Very potent marijuana, short for "Acapulco Gold"

Goof Balls - Barbiturates

Goon - PCP

Gorilla Pills - Tuinal (amobarbital sodium and secobarbital sodium)

Green - Dexamyl (dextroamphetamine sulfate and amobarbital) tablets/capsules. Low grade marijuana from Mexico

Green Hearts - Dexamyl (dextroamphetamine sulfate and amobarbital) tablets, 5 mg each

Greenies - Dexamyl (dextroamphetamine sulfate and amobarbital) tablets/capsules

Gun - Hypodermic needle used to inject drugs

Gutter - Vein used to inject drugs

Hard Candy - Heroin. By extension, any "hard" drugs

Harry - Heroin

Hearts - Three-sided, heart-shaped amphetamine tablets

Heaven Dust - Cocaine

Heavenly Gates - Morning glory seeds

Hog - PCP

Hog - Chloral hydrate

Hootch - Marijuana

Hooter - Marijuana

Horn - To sniff a drug

Horse Hearts - Benzedrine (amphetamine sulfate) tablets

Horse, Skag - Heroin

Horse Tranquilizer - PCP

Ice Cream Habit - Irregular drug habit

Incentive - Cocaine

J - Marijuana

Jellies - Chloral hydrate

Jelly Beans - Ethchlorvynol

Killer Weed - PCP mixed with marijuana and smoked

Kool-Aid - LSD mixed with punch

Krystal - PCP in solid form. Amphetamine in solid form

Lady Snow - Cocaine

Leaper - Amphetamine, no specific brand

Licorice Drops - Morning glory seeds

Lightning - Amphetamine, no specific brand

Lilly - Seconal (secobarbital)

Line - Short for "mainline." A vein used to inject drugs

Ludes - Quaaludes

Luding Out - Using methaqualone, either Quaalude or Sopor. Using methaqualone, either Quaalude or Sopor, with alcohol, usually wine.

Magic Mist - PCP

Master Greenjeans - Ethchlorvynol

Merck - General term for high-grade drugs

Mesc - Mescaline

Mexican Brown - Heroin of average strength

Mexican Red - Red capsules imported from Mexico, reported to contain secobarbital

Mexican Yellows - Phenobarbital, possibly Nembutal, possibly imported from Mexico

Mickies - LSD

Miss Emma - Morphine

Moon - Mescaline

Movie Star Drug - Cocaine

Mr. Natural - LSD

Nail - Hypodermic needle used to inject drugs

Nose Candy - Cocaine

Orange Hearts - Dexedrine (dextroamphetamine sulfate) tablets

Paris 400 - Parest (methaqualone hydrochloride) capsules, usually 400 mg each

Peace Pill - PCP

Pearly Gates - Morning glory seeds

Peyote - Mescaline

Pickles - Ethychlorvynol

Pimp - Cocaine

Pinks - Seconal (secobarbital) capsules. Darvon (propoxyphene hydrochloride) capsules

Pink Ladies - Seconal (secobarbital) capsules

Poppers - Amyl nitrite

Porker - PCP

Pumpkin Seeds - Benzodiazepines

Purple Haze - LSD in tablet form. PCP in purple tablet form

Quaas - Quaalude (methaqualone)

Reds and Greys - Darvon (propoxyphene

hydrochloride) capsules

Rippers - General term for amphetamines

Roches - Benzodiazepines

Rock - Cocaine in solid form

Rockets - Marijuana

Rocket Fuel - PCP

Roses - Benzedrine (amphetamine suflate) tablets

714s - Quaaludes

Sherman's - PCP cigarette

Short Flight - Combination of Coricidin (aspirin, chlorpheniramine maleate, and caffeine) and beer

Smack - Heroin

Snapper - Amyl nitrite

Snort - Inhale cocaine or heroin

Society High - Cocaine

Speed - Amphetamine

Speedball - Combination of amphetamine and cocaine or heroin for injection

Stardust - Cocaine

Strawbery Mescaline - Reddish-brown powder, reported to contain mescaline

Superjoint - Marijuana mixed with PCP for smoking

Super Quaalude - Sopor, Quaas, Ludes-Parest (methaqualone hydrochloride)

Tees and Blues (Tops and Bottoms) - Talwin and triplennamine

Tecata - Heroin

Texas Reefer - Long, fat, marijuana cigarette, also called a "bomber"

THC - tetrahydrocannabinol, possibly PCP

Thai Stick - Asian marijuana mixed with opium and tied to a reed

Tie Stick - Marijuana mixed with opium and tied to a popsicle stick

Toot - Cocaine

Tranks - Benzodiazepines

Truck Drivers - Amphetamines

Uncle Milties - Meprobamate

Water - Methamphetamine mixed with water for injection

Weed - Marijuana

Weekend Habit - Irregular drug use

Weekend Warrior - Irregular drug user

White Cross - Amphetamine tablets, from illicit manufacturers, which are white, and double scored

White Dexies - Amphetamine tablets from illicit manufacturers

White Girl - Cocaine

White Horizon - PCP

White Horse - Cocaine

White Stuff - Heroin, cocaine, morphine

Window Pane - LSD

Wobble - PCP

Yellow Ban - Methamphetamine, possibly Desoxyn

Yellow Jackets - Barbiturates

Zeeters - Amphetamines

Zip - Amphetamine

K. Suicide Attempts

1. Suicides rank as one of the leading causes of death in adolescents.
2. Suicide attempts (parasuicides) outnumber completed suicides by 10-150:1. The male-female suicide ratio is 5:1.
3. Both suicides and suicide attempts (parasuicides) can increase after media reporting of a real or fictional suicide vicitm. Clustering of suicides has occurred in certain communities.
4. Completed suicide attempts are more common in males; frequently, violent measures, often firearms, are used.
5. Suicide attempts are more common in females; frequently, ingestions (self-poisoning) are used.
6. Adolescents with chronic conditions can attempt suicide by self-poisoning through overdoses of their medications (e.g., theophylline) or neglecting

to take medications (e.g., insulin).

7. Although an acute event may trigger the suicide act, the following predisposing factors are common:

    a. Parental loss/broken home.
    b. Depression (tearfulness vs a raging "acting-out").
    c. Few friends/social supports.
    d. Failure socially or scholastically.
    e. Association with other troubled youth.
    f. Previous history of suicide gestures (very important!).
    g. A history of substance abuse or psychosocial problems not included above.

8. When a child or adolescent presents with suicidal behavior, take it very seriously!

9. Important historical information includes:

    a. Method used (type and number of pills, weapon, etc.) and time employed.
    b. Whether victim announced the act.
    c. Whether victim expresses a wish to die, feels hopeless, has a desire to try again (determine if patient has access to method and a plan for its use already worked out), or shows remorse about the attempt.
    d. The precipitating incident prior to the present attempt.
    e. Whether the patient has a past history of suicide attempts, depression, aggression/acting-out, drug/alcohol abuse, psychiatric illness.
    f. Whether there is a family history of psychiatric illness or suicide.
    g. The patient's interpersonal relationships with his parents, siblings, and friends.
    h. The patient's functioning in school.
    i. The patient's social support systems.

10. A complete PE is mandatory with particular emphasis on the skin (needle tracks, marks of inflicted injury), neurologic, and psychiatric assessments.

11. Depending on the method of the attempt, different treatments will be necessary (e.g., suturing lacerations, gastric emptying for ingestions, hyperbaric O_2 for CO poisoning, etc.).
12. An adolescent who has distanced himself from family and friends, disposed of valued possessions, talked about death or suicide, expressed hopelessness about the future, left a suicide note, or has attempted suicide violently (firearms, hanging, CO exposure) is at extremely high risk for a successful suicide in the future. Individual and family psychotherapy will be necessary.
13. Involvement as soon as possible by social work and psychiatry is mandatory.
14. Interviews with family members should be conducted.
15. Admission to either a medical or a psychiatric unit is advisable.

REFERENCES

Chest pain
1. Brenner J, Berman M: Chest pain in childhood and Adolescence. *J Adol Hth Care* 1983; 3:271-6.
2. Pantell R, Goodman B: Adolescent chest pain - A prospective study. *Pediatr* 1983; 71:881-7.
3. Perry L: Pinpointing the cause of pediatric chest pain. *Contemp Pediatr* 1985; 2:71-96.
4. Selbest S: Chest pain in children. *Pediatr* 1985; 75:1068-70.
5. Selbest S: Evaluation of chest pain in children. *Pediatr in Rev* 1986; 8:56-62.

Failure to Thrive
1. Chatoor I, et al: Non-organic failure to thrive . *Pediatr Ann* 1984; 13:829-50.
2. Goldbloom R: Growth failure in infancy. *Pediatr in Rev* 1987; 9:57-61.
3. Rosenn D, et al: Differentiation of organic from non-Organic failure to thrive syndrome in infancy. *Pediatr* 1980; 66:698-704.
4. Sills R, Sills I: Don't overlook environmental causes of Failure to thrive. *Contemp Pediatr* 1986; 3:25-42.
5. Sills R: Failure to Thrive. *AJDC* 1978; 132:967-9.

Hypertension
1. Bailie M, et al: Hypertension - more than ever, a pediatric concern. *Contemp Pediatr* 1985; 2:30-57.
2. Bailie M, et al: Hypertension - finding a safe and effective therapy. *Contemp Pediatr* 1985; 2:93-106.
3. Daniels S, et al: Clinical spectrum of intrinsic renovascular hypertension in children. *Pediatr* 1987; 80:698-704.
4. Goldring D, Hernandez A: Hypertension in children. *Pediatr in Rev* 1982; 03:235-46.
5. Ingelfinger J: Newer strategies for diagnosis and treatment of hypertension in childhood and adolescence. *Res & Staff Physic* 1984; 30:40-50.
6. Lieberman E: Hypertension in childhood and adoelscence *CIBA* clinical symposia. Vol. 30, #3, 1978.
7. Task Force on Blood Pressure Control in Children: Report of the second task force on blood pressure control in children-1987. *Pediatr* 1987; 79:125.

Joint Pain/Swelling
1. Barton LL, Dunkle LM, Habib FH: Septic arthritis in childhood: A 13 year review. *Am J Dis Child* 1987; 141:898-900.
2. Biro F, Gewanter HL, Baum J: The hypermobility syndrome. *Pediatr.* 1983; 72:701-706.
3. Brewer EJ Jr: Pitfalls in the diagnosis of juvenile rheumatoid arthritis. *Pediatr Clin N Am* 1986; 33:1015-1032.
4. Eichenfield AH: Diagnosis and management of Lyme disease. *Pediatr Ann* 1986; 15:583-592.
5. Kummanno I, Kallio P, Pelkonen P, et al: Clinical signs and laboratory tests in the differential diagnosis of arthritis in children. *Am J Dis Child* 1987; 141:34-40.
6. McCarthy PL, Wasserman D, Spiesel SZ, et al: Evaluation of arthritis and arthralgia in the pediatric patient. *Clin Pediatr* 1980; 19:183-190.
7. Schaller JG: Arthritis in children. *Pediatr Clin N Am* 1986; 33:1565-1579.
8. Schaller JG: Arthritis as a presenting manifestation of malignancy in children. *J Pediatr* 1972; 81:793-796.
9. Steere AC, Green J, Schoen RT, et al: Successful parenteral penicillin therapy of established Lyme arthritis. *NEJM* 1985; 312:869-874.
10. Steere AC, Malawista SE, Bartenhagen NH, et al: The clinical spectrum and treatment of Lyme disease. *Yale J Biol Med* 1984; 57:453-461.

Mucocutaneous lymph node syndrome
1. Crowley D: Cardiovascular complications of mucocutaneous lymph node syndrome. *PCNA* 1984; 31:1321-9.
2. Fatica N, et al: Detection and management of cardiac involvement in the Kawasaki syndrome. *Pediatr Ann* 1987; 16:639-43.
3. Hicks RV, Melish M: Kawasaki syndrome. *Pediatr Clin N Amer* 1986; 33:1151-1175.
4. Jacobs J: Management strategies in Kawasaki disease. *Pediatr Ann* 1986; 15:621-7.
5. Kato H, Inoue O, Akagi T: Kawasaki disease: cardiac problems and management. *Pediatr in Rev* 1987; 9:209-217.

6. Koren G, et al: Probable efficacy of high-dose salicylates in reducing coronary involvement in Kawasaki disease. *JAMA* 1985; 254:767-9.
7. Melish M: Kawasaki syndrome (mucocutaneous lymph node syndrome). *Pediatr in Rev* 1980; 2:107-114.
8. Morens D, et al: National surveillance of Kawasaki disease. *Pediatr* 1980; 65:21-5
9. Newburger J, et al: The treatment of Kawasaki syndrome with intravenous gamma globulin. *NEJM* 1986; 315:341-7.

Lymphadenopathy
1. Bedross AA, Mann JP: Lymphadenopathy in children. *Adv Pediatr* 1981; 28:341.
2. Kew LK, Stottmeier K, Sherman I, et al: Mycobacterial cervical lymphadenopathy: relation of etiologic agents to age. *JAMA* 1984; 251:1286.
3. Knight PJ, Mulne AF, Vassy LE. When is lymph node biopsy indicated in children with enlarged peripheral nodes? *Pediatrics* 1982; 69:391-396.
4. Margileth A. Cervical adenitis. *Pediatr in Rev* 1985; 7:13.
5. Slap GB, Brooks JJ, Schwartz JS. When to perform biopsies of enlarged peripheral lymph nodes in young patients. *JAMA* 1984; 252:1321-1326.

Myositits
1. Dietzman DE, Schaller JG, Ray CG, et al.: Acute myositis associated with influenza B infection. *Pediatr* 1976; 57:255.

Reye's Syndrome
1. Dezateux CA, Dinwiddie R, Helms Pe, et al: Recongition and early management of Reye's syndrome. *Arch Dis Child* 1986; 61:647-651.
2. Consensus Conference. Diagnosis and treatment of Reye's syndrome. *JAMA* 1981; 246:2441-2444.
3. Huggenloeher PR, Trauner DA: Reye's syndrome in infancy. *Pediatr* 1978; 62:84.
4. Rockoff MA, Pascucci RC: Reye's syndrome. *Emerg Med Clin North Am* 1983; 1:87-100.
5. Shaywitz BA, Rothstein P, Venes JL: Monitoring and management of increased intracranial pressure in Reye's syndrome: results in 29 children. 1980; 66:198-204.
6. Trauner DA: Reye's syndrome. *Curr Prob Pediatr* 1982; 12:1.

Stinging Insect Reactions
1. Graft DF, Schuberth KC: Hymenoptera allergy in children. *PCNA* 1983; 30:873.
2. Macguire JF, Geha RS: Bee, wasp, and hornet stings. *Pediatr in Rev* 1986; 8:5-11.
3. Valentine MD: Insect venom allergy: diagnosis and treatment. *J Allergy Clin Immunol* 1984; 73:299.

Substance Abuse
1. Felter R, Izsak, Lawrence HS. Emergency department management of the intoxicated adolescent. *Pediatr Clin North Am* 1987; 34:399.
2. Giannini AJ, Price WA, Giannini MC. Contemporary drugs of abuse. *American Family Practice* 1986; 33:207.
3. Kulberg A: Substance abuse: clinical identification and management. *Pediatr Clin North Am* 1986; 33:325-361.
4. McDonald DI: Drugs, drinking, and adolescence. *Amer J Dis Child* 1984; 138:117.
5. McHugh MJ. The abuse of volatile substances. *Pediatr Clin North Am* 1987; 34:333.
6. Meeks J: Adolescents at risk for drug and alcohol abuse. *Seminars Adoles Med* 1985; 1:231.
7. Treatment of acute drug abuse reactions. *Medical Letter* 1987; 29:83.
8. Zarek D, Hawkins D, Rogers PD. Risk factors for adolescent substance abuse. *PCNA* 1987; 34:481.

Suicide Attempts
1. Christoffel K, et al: Adolescent suicide and suicide attempts. *Pediatr Emerg Care* 1988; 4:32-40.
2. Committee on Adolescence: Suicide and suicide attempts in adolescents and young adults. *Pediatr* 1988; 81:322-4.
3. Eisenberg L: The epidemiology of adolescent suicide. *Pediatr Ann* 1984; 13:47-54.
4. Hergenroeder A, et al: The pediatrician's role in adolescent suicide. *Pediatr Ann* 1984; 13:787-98.
5. Pfeffer C: Clinical aspects of childhood suicidal behavior. *Pediatr Ann* 1984; 13:56-61.
6. Robbins D, Conroy R: A cluster of adolescent suicide attempts. *J Adol Hlth Care* 1983; 3:253-5.

Index

A